These Special Children

THESE SPECIAL CHILDREN

The Ostomy Book for

Parents

of Children with

Colostomies,

Ileostomies, and

Urostomies

BY *Katherine F. Jeter, Ed.D., E.T.*

ILLUSTRATIONS BY *John R. Jeter Jr.*

BULL PUBLISHING COMPANY, Palo Alto, California

TO JOHN—
Before the Phoenix, the genesis.

Copyright 1982
Bull Publishing Co.
Box 208, Palo Alto, CA 94302
(415) 322-2855

ISBN 0-915950-51-0

Manufactured in the United States of America

Foreword

The impact of a medical experience for a child depends to a great extent on how the parents and medical team deal with that child. It is not only essential for children to be prepared in advance for surgical procedures but they require a supportive adult who is sufficiently "askable" for the child to feel free to ask questions and have honest answers returned. My experience as a Pediatric Psychologist tells me that the most cooperative children, and those who respond positively to medical treatment, are ones who feel they've been treated honestly and respectfully by the health team. Clearly, emotional adjustment plays a very important role in the child's recovery. Moreover, a person's attitude toward their continued health care in adulthood is markedly influenced by how they were treated by adult professionals in childhood.

I've been called upon many times to assist parents and physicians in dealing with children who are about to receive an ostomy. Without any doubt, this book would have been ideal as an aide to help parents and children.

I am convinced that this book should be a document made available to every physician, nurse and health professional who deals with children as surgical patients.

LEE SALK, PH.D.

Contents

Acknowledgments

To the surgeons: Dr. John Kingsley Lattimer, and Drs. Robert Bertsch, Dudley Danoff, John Duckett, Richard Ehrlich, Rainer Engel, Clarence Hewitt, Thomas Santulli, Gilbert Simon, John Schullinger, and Myron Roberts;

To the Children: John, Vicky, Joey, Kristy, Sid (who used to be Sidney), David, Richie, Amy, and several hundred more;

To the parents: Judy and Neil, Roberta and Curt, Pam and Harlan, and dear Mrs. Soan—who represent the heartache and triumph of all parents who are called upon to be supermen and superwomen around the clock for years and years—

THEY WERE MY CLINICAL INSTRUCTORS

To the professors: Drs. Frank Krause, Gary Lawson, and Donna Pearre in Ball State University's European program; Drs. Gloria Horrworth, Donald Linkowski, Salvatore Paratore, Martha Rashid, Daniel Sinick, and Clemmont Vontress at The George Washington University—

THEY ADDED SCHOLARSHIP

To Donald P. Binder and The United Ostomy Association who asked me to write and Bull Publishing who saw the importance of publishing;

To Al and Agnes Evans, Duke Nauton, Marge Peterson, Kathy Biggs, and Lois Corti, RN, MPH, ET for their particular contributions and sustained encouragement;

To Barbara Torbert whose typewriter met every deadline and whose quiet efficiency made working with the manuscript so easy;

To John R. Jeter, Jr., the menderer and artist, and our people—Sally, John, and Stephen—

THEY HAVE BEEN CATALYSTS, PROMOTERS,
AND VALUED ASSISTANTS

And, most recently,

Drs. Lawrence Winkler of The George Washington University School of Education, Dr. Harry Miller of The George Washington University School of Medicine, and Dr. Mary Robinson of The Children's Hospital National Medical Center whose enthusiasm for and attention to this project amplified its scope immeasurably.

A COMPROMISE

Grammarians may shudder at the incorrect use of "ostomies" when most children have only one. Parents may feel that the plural "they" and "them" is impersonal. The choice was to use singular pronouns and to choose between the sexes or switch awkwardly from "he" to "she."

   It seemed more comfortable to speak to parents and children collectively; to talk about doctors and nurses as a group; and to discuss ostomies in general than to use singular and, sometimes, sexist language. Thank you for understanding.

Preface

Ostomy is an unusual word. It is not in the dictionary; not many people are sure exactly what it means, but most are certain they don't want one! An ostomy is a surgically formed opening. The ostomies we are talking about are surgically formed openings in the gastrointestinal or urinary systems to allow for the elimination of body wastes—stool or urine.

Twenty years ago is ancient history in the field of ostomy care. Few people had heard of ostomies. Even fewer had seen or heard of a child with an ostomy. Many nurses finished their training without having cared for a patient with one. There were only one or two appliances small enough for pediatric patients. There were no certified enterostomal therapists (ETs), and there was nothing that parents of a child ostomate could read that explained the special care the child and the ostomy would require.

In only two decades there have been many advances. Most people have heard at least something about ostomies, even if they aren't aware that children have them. Rolf Benirschke, a place kicker for a professional football team, had an ileostomy in 1980 and returned to help his team, the San Diego Chargers, nearly make it to Super Bowl XV. A South African magazine reported in April 1980 that Petula Clark, the pop singer, has an ileostomy. Many of the Poster Children for the National Foundation have had ostomies.

Now there are many child-size appliances and accessories available. Nurses learn more than they used to about the physical care, and the psychological rehabilitation after ostomy, and there are 1135 certified ETs, who are registered nurses especially trained to care for patients with ostomies.

Missing still, however has been a resource book that could be given to parents of children who need ostomies—a book that would inform, counsel and comfort. This book is intended to do those three things.

Where has the information been gathered? It has come from twenty years of clinical experience with child ostomates and their parents; youth "rap sessions"; parent support groups; formal research projects; review of the scientific literature; hundreds of interviews; and from families who have written from all over the United States and abroad, seeking or offering assistance. And it comes from years of postgraduate study of child and adolescent development and counseling.

October, 1981   Katherine Jeter

Introduction

Why This Book

Children are special people. They are special because they are not, as artists portrayed them in the 1800s, miniature adults. Their emerging personalities are products of their genetic inheritance and their experiences.

Their ability to understand what is happening to them, to solve problems, and to express themselves changes as they mature. Children don't just "know more" when they are seven than they did when they were three. They "know differently." For these reasons it is important to understand how children's minds, bodies, personalities, and emotions are shaped in order to promote effective social and intellectual growth. When children are born with deformities, or acquire diseases that interfere with average activities of growing up, their special needs must be considered—in addition to the usual needs of every child.

Ostomies are special conditions. They are not illnesses or diseases in themselves, but they require special care—particular appliances and accessories, special plans for school or travel, and regular attention, to prevent unnecessary complications and to deal with those that are unavoidable.

Parenting is now recognized as a challenge in itself. In recent years family planning has become more precise, and more attention has been given to helping men and women prepare for their roles as parents. There are prepared childbirth classes. The sight of expectant couples leaving the hospital with their quilts and pillows, chattering about labor stages and breathing exercises, is a pleasant contrast to the earlier tradition of mothers being wheeled through closed doors while pacing fathers waited to learn what their wives had delivered them. There are neighborhood meetings for new mothers, family and parents groups in community centers, and programs for single parents.

Many parents of children with deformities or illnesses have said they don't "fit in" to these programs, that their concerns are special and go beyond what other families want to discuss. Parents of children with ostomies are required to learn more about bodily systems and functions than most people ever want or need to know. They must learn to converse in a new language—about electrolytes and urine pH, face plates and tail closures, IVPs and colonoscopy. They also should learn as much as they can about average childhood milestones, so they will have a yardstick by which to measure their own children's progress or delays. When parents are alert to stresses that commonly arise where children are ill, sometimes between parents, sometimes among brothers and sisters resentful of the special attention to another, they can take steps to avoid additional unhappiness, and to ease tensions before they get out of hand.

It is not enough, then, to offer a pamphlet just about ostomies, or about why ostomies are performed in childhood, or which appliances are best for which age and kind of ostomy. Children are special people, and these are special children, with many problems common to all and some unique to themselves. Likewise you, their parents, will experience many of the joys and frustrations common to parents everywhere; but you also are sure to discover depths of sadness and heights of accomplishment that are yours alone.

This IS an ostomy book for parents, but it is also a book to help parents understand that a child ostomate is, at all times, first a child.

How to Use This Book

Most of the information in this book should be useful for all parents of young ostomates. But there will be special interest in those parts which deal with your particular problems—your child's physical disabilities and type of ostomy, your child's particular interests and needs at different times, your family's particular strengths and weaknesses. So you will want to be able to move around in the book, looking things up, and reading what is of greatest interest at the particular time.

You will probably want to skip ahead to Section V, "Conditions That Lead to Ostomies," and read at least the part dealing with your child's condition. Specific parts of Section I, relating to your child's ostomy, will have more meaning than the rest of that section, and the succeeding three sections dealing with children at different stages of development and various groups that relate to them, will have different usefulness and meaning at different times. You should have regular recourse to the "Frequently Asked Questions," lists of "Resources," descriptions of "Appliances" and "Aids," and to the Glossary, as appropriate.

You should make note of the "Drawings for Children," beginning on p. 176; these are intended for coloring in, to help make learning about bodies, ostomy operations, and ostomy care a positive and natural part of your child's experience. Also the general anatomical drawings on pp. 3, 100–2 should be of recurring interest, as you become familiar with why, where and how all of this is happening.

Of course any author hopes that readers will want to sit down and read the book straight-through (and is somewhat perplexed as to why some don't). But whether or not that happens, ultimately the major part of what is presented here should be of interest and use to you.

Finally, we hope that this book will initiate a sharing process—that you will share with us and ultimately with others what you learn. So take to heart the message on p. 168. We look forward to hearing from you.

Ostomies Explained

How They Are Alike

Ostomy, means a surgically created opening. The word ostomy really is a suffix; but since people with ostomies began getting together to help one another in 1949 in Philadelphia, the suffix has become a handy and accepted word to use when generalizing. The location of the ostomy is specified by the prefix: *colo-* tells you the opening is in the colon; *ileo-*, in the ileum or small intestine, etc.

Stoma means mouth. It is common to refer to the nipple of exposed intestine or urinary organ as the stoma. To be perfectly accurate, stoma should refer only to the opening itself; but now is not the time to change the tide of popular usage, so in this book, stoma also will refer generally to the portion of tissue that is brought out on the abdomen or flank.

Most stomas are red (like the lining of the mouth or nose), because they are actually mucous membrane. They bleed easily if they are nicked with a fingernail or brushed by a bath towel or gauze pad, because there is no skin covering the thousands of vessels and capillaries. Bleeding usually stops as quickly as it starts. When it does not, ice may be applied. If it persists, of course, the doctor should be notified. As raw and sore as a stoma appears, it has no feeling because there are no nerve endings in the exposed organ. It is difficult to believe that stomas are not easily injured in childhood activity, but they rarely are. Generally speaking, stomas may be slept on, rolled on, and even sat upon by another child for a few minutes, without undue concern.

Parents often are frightened by their first sight of a stoma. So are young children. Older children may respond with "Oh, Yuk!" and be repelled at the first glimpse of their new body part.

Stomas are a living organ with a regular peristaltic (rythmic contracting) movement. Once children have gotten used to the fact of their stoma, they may be absolutely fascinated by its constant motion.

An ostomy requires particular care, but the stoma itself needs little more than a clean environment. A stoma does not need to be washed; but on the other hand it is perfectly fine to put a child into the bathtub or shower without an appliance or stomal covering. (The only exception to this is pyelostomies and nephrostomies, which will be discussed later.) Bathwater does not enter the stoma because of the constant outward peristaltic action.

Stomas do not become infected as you think of a cut or abrasion becoming infected. What happens is that they can become ulcerated, if they are in constant contact with an irritating appliance, or, in the case of urinary stomas, they can become encrusted and inflamed if they are over-run with bacteria in appliances that are encrusted with urinary sediment.

Surgeons know a lot about constructing stomas. Enterostomal therapists (ETs) and other trained specialists know a great deal about managing them. But in a few short weeks of on-the-job training parents become the undisputed authorities on their own children's ostomy. No one will ever know as much about this one stoma as you do.

You do not need a college degree, or even a high school diploma, to become a skilled technician in ostomy care. But it is important that you take advantage of all the teaching offered and learn as much as you possibly can, even if it's just one new piece of information per week. As you gain knowledge you will be able to recognize subtle change that may signal trouble around the corner; you will gain confidence in your ability to make decisions that affect the quality of your child's life; and you will win the respect and appreciation of doctors and nurses who want you to become an active part of the health care team. Children with ostomies need informed parents to serve as their advocates.

An ostomy is not a disease or an illness. This deserves restatement. By itself an ostomy with an appliance should not restrict employment, academic success, or social pleasure; but of course, there cannot ever be "just an ostomy." There is a birth defect, a disease, or an injury that came first. And that will be a distinctive part of your childs' experience. But there is much more that will make the child's care unique. NEVER-TO-BE-FORGOTTEN, there is a person behind every ostomy—a person with a cultural heritage and a distinctive personality that will determine how much can be accepted and how much accomodated.

What about children? They are very much at the mercy of their cultural inheritance. Their personalities are in the process of development, and will become the sum of their biological, psychological, and social experiences. Their attitude toward feces and urine, toward the alteration of body function, and about their illness—their whole image of themselves will be affected by what they see and hear first from their parents, and then from health professionals, neighbors, playmates and relatives. Understanding ostomy care and taking it in stride is a positive step toward healthy acceptance and psychological wellbeing.

The discussion of ostomies that follows is not meant to be fully digested in an afternoon. There is a new language to be learned. (You will find the Glossary in Section IX helpful.)

How They Are Different

Each ostomy is done for a different purpose, and each functions in a particular manner that will determine the care it requires and the equipment that is used.

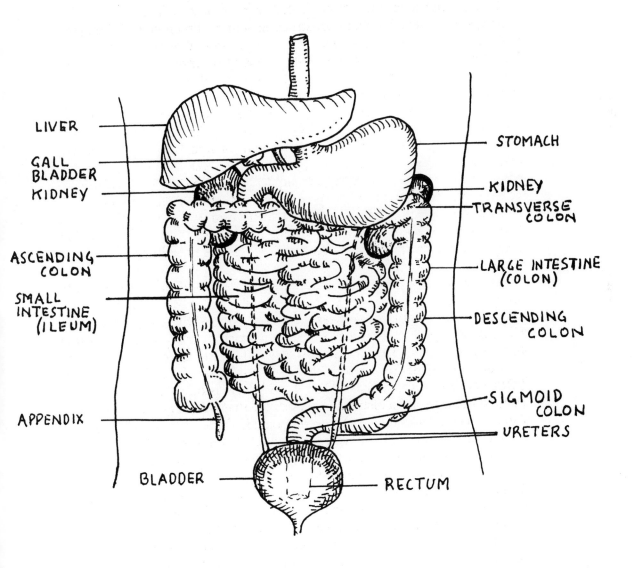

LIVER

GALL
BLADDER

KIDNEY

ASCENDING
COLON

SMALL
INTESTINE
(ILEUM)

APPENDIX

BLADDER

STOMACH

KIDNEY

TRANSVERSE
COLON

LARGE INTESTINE
(COLON)

DESCENDING
COLON

SIGMOID
COLON

URETERS

RECTUM

FIGURE 1   GASTROINTESTINAL AND URINARY ORGANS

How Colostomies Are Constructed

The colon has been described as a transporter, water absorber, and storage compartment. A colostomy may be created in the ascending, transverse, descending, or sigmoid colon. (Figure 1) (Since there is but a small distance between the descending and sigmoid colon, the two will be considered together in the following discussion.)

Looking at an ASCENDING COLOSTOMY on the right side of the body (we will refer to the ostomate's "right" and "left"), you can visualize that stool hasn't gone very far from the small intestine, so not much water or minerals have been absorbed. (Figure 2) There are likely to be plenty of digestive enzymes left in the feces at this point. These enzymes can't distinguish between body waste and skin. It takes only a few hours for them to "digest" normal skin tissue, leaving a red, painful weeping mess behind. Children's sensitive skin cannot stand confrontation with such an enemy, and it is important for this reason to use a skin barrier (an application, sometimes in the form of a wafer around the stoma protecting the skin—see Glossary).

The stool probably will be about the consistency of toothpaste, but may be only thick liquid (resembling a milk shake) when solid food is restricted.

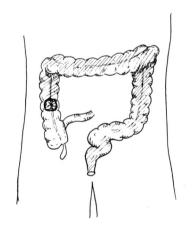

FIGURE 2 ASCENDING COLOSTOMY

When there is no reason to remove the colon to the left of (farther along the digestive tract beyond) the colostomy, some provision must be made for it. The surgeon may make a loop colostomy in the ascending colon, or a divided or double-barrel colostomy. Even though there really are two stomas in a loop colostomy, after a month or so the nonfunctioning stoma may be hardly noticeable. In the divided or double-barrel colostomy, stool will come out of the right-hand stoma but only mucus will come from the other one.

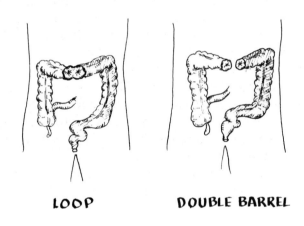

LOOP   DOUBLE BARREL

FIGURE 3   TRANSVERSE COLOSTOMY

The resting portion of the colon is still very much alive. It will be secreting mucus; there may be some old residue left in it; and in a loop colostomy, fecal material may even spill over into it. It may be necessary to gently flush it by putting warm tap water or normal saline (water with salt in it) into the stoma and allowing it to be passed through the anus (but ONLY if the physician ordered it). Older children will be able to tell you that they feel like they need to have a bowel movement. This is perfectly normal and many times they are able to expel something when they sit on the toilet.

A TRANSVERSE COLOSTOMY (Figure 3) will function much like a colostomy from the ascending colon. Usually it is constructed either as a loop or divided colostomy. A transverse colostomy generally is created to rest or protect the colon below it and may not be required for too long, maybe several months or a year. The stool is rarely formed, but it may be thicker than the stool from a right-sided colostomy simply because it has passed over more absorptive bowel surface before reaching the stoma and leaving the body.

When children have a DESCENDING or SIGMOID COLOSTOMY (Figure 4) most of the colon is functioning, so the stool is nearly the consistency it would be if it came from the rectum. The rectum may or may not require removal, depending on the underlying reason for the colostomy. Removal of the rectum is called *proctectomy*. As long as any portion of the colon and the rectum are intact, remember that there may be normal feelings of the urge to have a bowel movement.

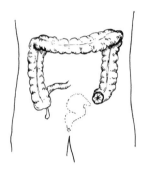

FIGURE 4   DESCENDING OR SIGMOID COLOSTOMY

If your child passes material in the diaper or underpants, or when sitting on the toilet, you need not be concerned unless there is bright red blood or signs of infection, such as pus or a putrid odor. (It is a good idea to have your surgeon describe to you the sort of discharge that is cause for concern.)

Because adults have more colostomies than ileostomies or urostomies, most ostomy literature is concerned with colostomies. Much of it deals with regulating sigmoid colostomies by means of irrigation—essentially an enema every day or two, which empties the bowel and reduces reliance on an appliance. Colostomies in children are not usually regulated. More often, they are managed with a throw-away saran or plastic pouch and a skin barrier*. (Some nurses and physicians believe that it is prefer-

---

*It is assumed in this book that parents will have begun to learn the techniques and products of ostomy management, almost from the moment of learning the need for an ostomy. For general reference, see the section on Products and Accessories, p. 151, and ask your physician, ET, or other professional for guidance to explanation literature.

able to cover the skin with ointments and dressings. Perhaps they have not seen the newer skin barriers such as Stomahesive and the small pouches made specially for children by several companies.)

Once the children are at home and their parents take charge, colostomy care is likely to be determined by

- Consistency and number of daily stools
- Convenience of washing facilities
- Availability of appliances

- Ease of application
- Time
- Cost

How They Are Managed

Sammie, Rachel and Kirk* are three babies who needed colostomies. Their mothers use different techniques; each believes her method to be the easiest and to require the least amount of time. All three children have excellent skin, with only occasional minor problems from diarrhea.

Sammie weighs 12 pounds. He has a right-sided colostomy and passes loose stool frequently. His mother, Mrs. T., uses Stomahesive® wafer (Squibb), a small saran pouch (Byram Surgical), and liquid ostomy soap (United). This is Mrs. T.'s method (See Figure 5):

Each morning at bathtime she washes the peristomal skin (the skin around the stoma) with ostomy soap on a non-sterile gauze pad, then rinses the skin well and pats it dry. She places a Stomahesive wafer, that she prepared earlier, around the ostomy. The inside "donut hole" diameter is ¾" and just fits to the base of the stoma. The outside diameter is 2". She applies the adhesive disc of the saran pouch to the Stomahesive wafer and uses a circular motion with her index finger up inside to bond pouch adhesive to Stomahesive and minimize possibility of wrinkles that would permit leakage. The adhesive on the saran pouch has the same dimensions, so only Stomahesive is against the skin. Occasionally she places two strips of hypoallergenic paper or pink plastic tape on either side of the adhesive area for added security. She empties the contents every three to four hours, sometimes using a little ear syringe with a small amount of warm water to wash out the stool. Mrs. T. folds the bottom of the pouch twice, pleats it across and wraps it several times with a small rubber band purchased from a stationery store in large quantities.

*All of the children described in this book are real people; only their names have been changed.

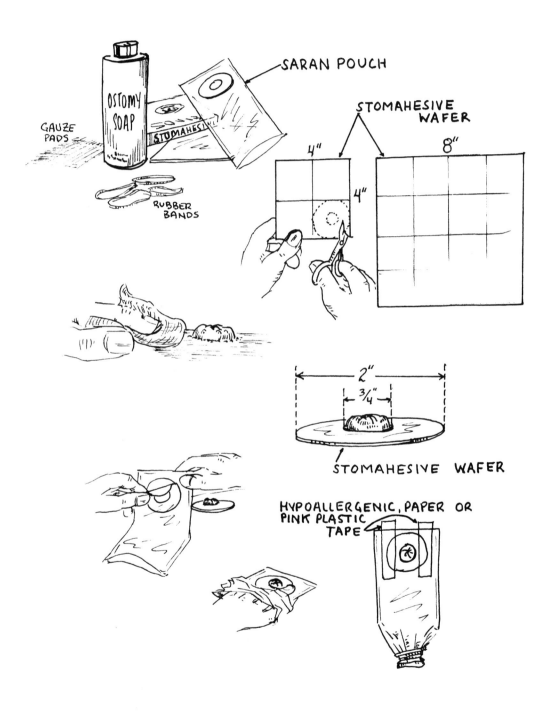

GAUZE PADS

OSTOMY SOAP

STOMAHES...

SARAN POUCH

RUBBER BANDS

STOMAHESIVE WAFER

4"

4"

8"

2"

3/4"

STOMAHESIVE WAFER

HYPOALLERGENIC, PAPER OR PINK PLASTIC TAPE

FIGURE 5   SAMMIE

Rachel's mother (Mrs. G.) uses another method. (See Figure 6) Rachel weighs 6½ pounds and was born with neonatal necrotizing enterocolitis (See p.103). She has a divided transverse colostomy but there is not enough room between the two

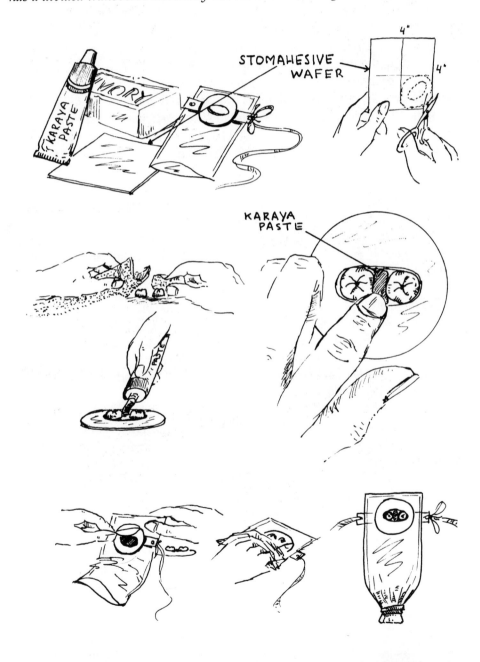

STOMAHESIVE WAFER

KARAYA PASTE

FIGURE 6   RACHEL

stomas to put a pouch over just the functioning one. The ET made a template (pattern) for Mrs. G. It measures 2" in diameter and the inside opening is cut in an oval to go around both stomas. Mrs. G. also uses Stomahesive. In addition she uses Ivory soap, a saran premie pouch (Byram), and Karaya Paste® (Hollister). After Mrs. G. washes Rachel's skin with Ivory and rinses off the soap residue, she pats it dry with the corner of a soft bath towel. Then she applies a wafer of Stomahesive that has been cut according to the template. Between the two stomas there is skin exposed. Here Mrs. G. puts a dab of Karaya Paste with her finger, making certain that there is no skin left showing, and gives the Paste time to dry until shiny. The pouch she uses has a soft flexible plastic piece (between the saran and the adhesive) called a retainer or a face plate. This face plate has a tab on either side with a hole in it to permit the use of a belt. Mrs. G. uses ribbon or twill tape the nurses gave her (sometimes referred to as "trach tape" because it is used with tracheostomies) to tie around Rachel's abdomen for added support. Usually Mrs. G. changes the pouch every second morning, but sometimes leakage requires that it be reapplied more frequently. She also finds an ear syringe handy for washing out thicker stool. She closes the pouch with a small stationery clip and then wraps a tissue or piece of gauze around it and secures it with a rubber band so the metal clip doesn't dig into the baby's skin.

Kirk's mother (Mrs. E.) scoffs at these two methods and says they sound like a lot of unnecessary time and trouble! She wasn't given any instruction in ostomy care when she took Kirk home from the hospital with one disposable diaper wrapped around his waist for the colostomy drainage and one between his legs for urine. She devised her own system (See Figure 7) and has had no cause to change it in the eight months she has been caring for her son.

Kirk now weighs 23 pounds. His colostomy is on the left side and he has three or four partially formed stools per day. Mrs. E. puts him in the bath tub each morning and washes him all over, including the peristomal skin around and up to the stoma, with "any old soap" in the bathroom. After his bath she drys this peristomal skin well and wipes it with Protective Barrier Film® (Bard). She covers a wide area, leaving a thin plastic film to protect the skin. (It is dry when it is slick to the touch and shiny in appearance.) Then she mixes a paste of zinc oxide ointment (from the drugstore) and karaya powder (from a surgical supplier) into a spreadable consistency about like peanut butter. She applies a generous coating of this paste in a circle around the stoma—about 2½". She cuts a facial tissue in a similar circular form with an opening to fit the ⅞" stoma. She places this tissue cover over the paste and pats it gently.

Mrs. E. diapers Kirk in the normal manner using disposable diapers. When he moves his bowels, she simply peels away tissue and stool and replaces a thin layer *of paste and new tissue circle. She only removes all the paste and "starts from scratch" in the morning, unless Kirk has been on medication or has a cold or flu that causes him to have more frequent loose stools that are irritating to his skin. Mr. E. is an expert in Kirk's care, too, and laughs when he admits that he never once changed his other children's diapers.*

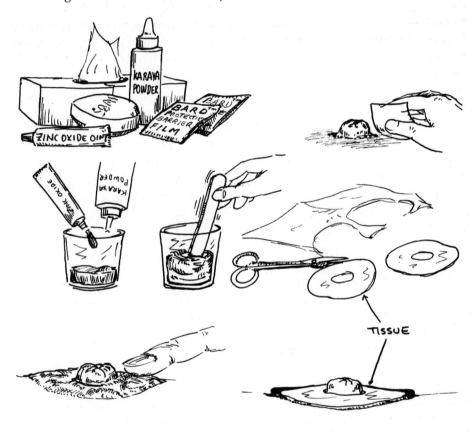

TISSUE

FIGURE 1   KIRK

All three mothers stress the importance of keeping the children clothed so they can't scratch their stomas or pull at the pouches and dislodge them. (Babies prefer appliances and their contents to all other crib toys, 2 to 1! When they are not wearing one-piece stretch terry jump suits, their undershirts should be pinned securely to their diapers.)

Sean and Tammy are older. (See Figure 8) Both go to school all day. Sean has a transverse colostomy with a nice round 1¼" stoma. Tammy's colostomy is in the descending colon and is ⅞" in diameter. Sean wears a Hollister Karaya Seal Drainable Stoma Bag® with Microporous Adhesive.® It is 12" long. He uses the closure clip that comes in the box. Usually Sean changes every other day unless he's been swimming a lot, the weather is very hot, or he's had particularly loose stools that cause the karaya ring to melt more rapidly than normal. Tammy prefers a closed Karaya Seal Stoma Bag® without any adhesive. Sometimes, she whispers, she can take it off, shake the formed stool in the toilet and replace it. When Tammy takes a shower after gym class, she tucks the pouch in her locker, puts her hand over the stoma, and gets under the shower like everyone else. Her closest friends know about her colostomy but she doesn't want to invite the curiosity of classmates she doesn't know well. Both kids feel more comfortable wearing a belt.

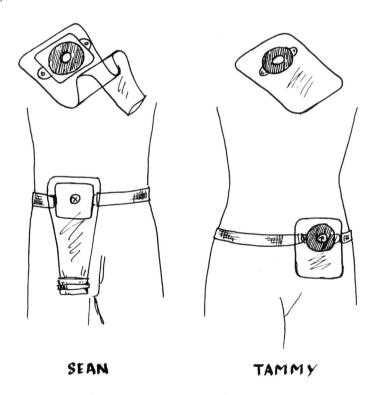

SEAN   TAMMY

FIGURE 8   COLOSTOMIES

Melanie is 13 and manages her colostomy as if it were an ileostomy. (See Figure 9) She met a lady at an ostomy association meeting, liked the method she used and tried it, and found it works well for her too. She uses a small karaya washer (Atlantic) around her stoma and a Mini-Flowered Extra Ileo B Pouch® (Coloplast). Sometimes she uses blue flowers; sometimes yellow. She always wears cotton underpants the same color as her pouch. Melanie uses tape around the adhesive edges like a picture frame and never wears a belt. She puts deodorant drops in each time she empties. She's lucky and only has to change her appliance twice a week. But, Melanie adds, this convenience only has come since she has become more careful about emptying the pouch and since her abdomen has grown. She showers daily and takes a bath "when the mood strikes."

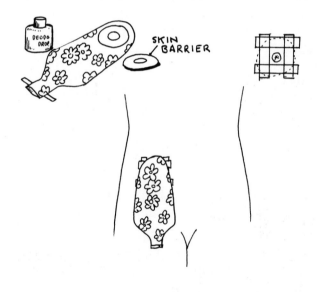

FIGURE 9   MELANIE

It might be safe to summarize techniques of care in this way: If all the children who had colostomies were gathered into one auditorium, there probably would be that many methods of management. The system doesn't matter as long as the child is comfortable, there is never any odor, the skin remains in excellent condition, and the procedure is affordable.

Colostomy Questions

■ Do colostomies smell?

Of course stool has an odor. (It will in part depend on many things, such as diet, medication, infection, etc.) But it should be completely controllable. There are preparations to be taken by mouth and deodorants to be put in the pouch. In addition, there are two rules that apply to every person, young and old, with a colostomy:

1. Cleanliness is important to good health and imperative to the prevention of embarrassing odors.

2. The colostomy pouch must be made with an odor barrier film. In this day and age there is no reason for any person, rich or poor, healthy or frail, to have a colostomy appliance that permits odor to pass through.

■ What about gas and noise?

In the absence of an anal sphincter the passage of gas cannot be controlled. It does make a noise and it is more noticeable because it comes from an opening on the abdomen instead of between the legs and ample folds of skin. Thankfully, the sound of passing gas is generally muffled by several layers of clothing. Some foods, like dried beans, cucumbers, etc., may contribute to gas. Chewing gum, an empty stomach, carbonated drinks, and swallowed air also contribute.

Immediately after bowel surgery most patients complain of a lot of gas, and everyone is more alert to it and nervous about it in the early weeks. The intestines should be expected to "settle down" after a regular diet and activity is resumed. If your child continues to be bothered by troublesome gas, there are numerous remedies offered in Ostomy Association newsletters and you may want to seek a doctor's advice.

DO NOT POKE A HOLE IN A COLOSTOMY POUCH TO LET GAS ESCAPE UNLESS YOU RESEAL IT WITH AN ADHESIVE PATCH

■ Will my child need a special diet?

Colostomies themselves do not require a special diet; but your child's associated conditions may necessitate food restrictions or cause food intolerances.

■ Must we irrigate our child's colostomy?

No. Irrigation is simply an enema or "wash out." A colostomy MUST be irrigated only when there is constipation or impaction that has been unresponsive to other measures. Otherwise irrigation is an investment in time made for the convenience of regulating bowel movements.

A good irrigation empties the entire colon. Stool that comes into the large intestine after the irrigation requires hours or days to make its way through the ascending and transverse colon. By the time it is ready to be passed through the stoma, another irrigation empties the entire intestine. Irrigation is a time-consuming method of colostomy regulation with which few parents and fewer children want to be bothered.

There are probably hundreds of other questions that already have or may soon pop into your mind. Write them down in the space provided in the back of the book. If they are not answered elsewhere in the book, you will have them to ask of your surgeon, an ET, or maybe the mother of another child with a colostomy.

How Ileostomies Are Constructed

ILEOSTOMIES bring the small intestine through the abdominal wall, bypassing the colon (large intestine). They are usually performed when the colon is so damaged by disease that good health and normal activity are being sacrificed. They present special challenges. (Without the water absorptive surface of the large intestine the patient has numerous loose stools daily.) But anyone, even children, can live comfortably without a colon—if some modifications in lifestyle are made.

There are two principal methods* that may be used to compensate when a colon must be removed. They are a conventional ileostomy, and most recently, a continent ileostomy.

CONVENTIONAL ILEOSTOMY

Reviewing the anatomy lesson (p. 4), when the colon is sacrificed it means that water and some minerals will not be absorbed, and there is no place for storage. (Figure 10)

---

*An additional alternative is the ileorectal anastamosis in which the surgeon puts the end of the small intestine into the rectum, eliminating the need for an ostomy.

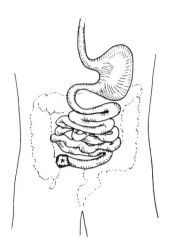

FIGURE 10   **ILEOSTOMY**

Pasty fecal material oozes from the stoma frequently during the day, with most of the activity occurring a little while after meals and less during the night. It is important to understand that there will not be formed or regular stools. (Some people report that, after they have had an ileostomy for some time, the end of the small intestine begins to act like a colon, absorbing liquid so that the stool becomes thicker.) An appliance must be worn at all times.

Fecal matter usually does not have an offensive odor as it leaves the small intestine, unless odor-producing foods such as onion, garlic or shellfish have recently been on the menu. Odor mounts as stool collects in the appliance. There are countless remedies. The many people with ileostomies—young and old—are living testimonies to their effectiveness, with no personal odor about themselves and no tell-tale odor when they leave a bathroom.

Most children who need an ileostomy have been very very sick. Either they have been sick for a long time with the warning symptoms of inflammatory bowel disease, and the continuous treatments with cortisone enemas, Azulfadine, and steroids; or they have become acutely and frighteningly ill with toxic megacolon*. As shocking as the concept of

---

Toxic means poison; *mega-* means large. The danger in this condition is that the colon will rupture (tear open) and spill infection inside the body.

having an ileostomy may be, and as much as some parents and children will resist the surgery, it provides dramatic relief when the cause is inflammatory bowel disease. Mrs. R. smiled as she recalled her daughter's surgery. She said, "I had been telling the doctors for months that we couldn't go on like we were. I was so frustrated that they didn't seem to be listening to me. Nevertheless, the day they came into the room and told us they would have to perform an ileostomy, I jumped up and said, "But she's not THAT sick!"

But despite the fears, young people who have had an ileostomy after suffering from inflammatory bowel disease would not exchange their ileostomy for the symptoms that led to it. Some say they wish they had not waited so long. Those are encouraging words for parents who dread making a crucial decision for their children.

When an ileostomy is being planned, the surgeon or an ET will examine their patient in all postural positions—sitting, squatting, jumping, bending, etc. It is absolutely essential to have a stoma on a smooth surface of the abdomen, away from skin folds, hip bones, scars, and existing or future pubic hair. It is not uncommon for youngsters to wear an appliance for several days before their operation to assist in locating the best site. The incision is usually down the midline or slightly to one side. The belly button is left undisturbed!

How They are Managed

A protruding nipple is created because patients have taught surgeons, by their experiences, that it is important to have a spout-effect into the appliance to minimize leakage and the painful skin irritation it causes. One mother lamented, "I thought Patty's flat stoma was so much nicer than the other children's I had seen UNTIL I found out how much more often we were changing her appliance." A stomal bud that protrudes ½" to 1" from the abdomen does not "stick out" under normal clothing. That is everyone's fear. If you are not convinced just because someone tells you that it's so, ask to meet another young person or adult who has had an ileostomy.

With this new method of elimination there are some noticeable differences. Hard-to-digest foods, such as corn and tomato skins, will exit the body looking remarkably as they did when they entered! Beets turn the stool beet red. This is not abnormal.

Obstruction of the ileostomy can, and does, occur. Some foods, like nuts and popcorn, are high on the list of those that cause trouble.

Dr. Victor Fazio, of the Cleveland Clinic, told a group of ETs that the Christmas holidays always seemed to be particularly busy in the Emergency Room with a dramatic rise in obstructed ileostomies. When children do not chew their food well and swallow large pieces, discomfort may be on its way. A gentle lavage (wash out) may be necessary to relieve the obstruction. This should NEVER be done without a doctor's advice. UNDER NORMAL CIRCUMSTANCES AN ILEOSTOMY IS NEVER IRRIGATED.

Food tolerance is an individual and sometimes a regional thing. Steve and Cindy are two particularly memorable teenagers. Steve had not been able to eat pizza for nearly two years before surgery because it aggravated his colitis so badly. Cindy, who was from the Southwest, had been on a bland diet for almost a year before her surgery. After their operations, both made up for lost time. Steve said "no thank you" to the mashed potatoes and pureed chicken that was to have been his first real meal after surgery and ordered out for a pizza. Cindy ate little else but enchiladas and tamales for weeks.

Much has been written about diet for the ostomate. It will be discussed with you in the hospital. (If the dietician is not sent to you, you are welcome to make an appointment to see her.) Generally speaking it is better to give children freedom to choose what they like to eat than to nag them with dozens of "not allowed" rules. Several mothers have confessed that it was very difficult to break away from the cooking routines they had established during their childrens' pre-surgery illnesses. After surgery it took a while for them to realize that the carefully prepared low-residue meals they had fixed each day were more satisfying to their own needs than their childrens'. Such admissions may be difficult, but they are progress toward restoring normalcy in a household.

Long hot baths may loosen the adhesvie seal of an appliance, but a bath should never be given up just to keep a pouch on for one more day. It is perfectly fine and desirable for children to take a bath without their appliance on. However, stooling in the shower or bath water may be upsetting to them.

The enzymes that are in the stool, and which can harm skin so rapidly, have been discussed earlier, but deserve a second mention. Complaining of burning, itching, and discomfort around the stoma is not "silly"; it is not "healing"; and it's not "being a sissy." Such complaints generally indicate that fecal drainage is seeping under the appliance face plate, and it is time to reexamine the seal protecting the skin. It is very important for skin up to the stoma to be covered with a skin barrier. The general rule for fitting the face plate is to allow ⅛" for the stoma to expand. (That is, a

1" stoma would require a 1⅛" opening for the face plate.) A skin barrier of some type is used to cover any exposed skin. Any of the gelatinous wafers may actually "hug" the stoma without harming it.

Just as with colostomy care, there are countless effective methods for managing an ileostomy. Shelly and Mike both had ileostomies for inflammatory bowel disease. Shelly had Crohn's disease and Mike had ulcerative colitis. Shelly is in junior high school and Mike is in high school. Their methods of management are quite different but both are satisfied with their routine and neither would want to try anything new at this time.

Shelly is 5'4" tall and weights 103 pounds. She has a lovely figure. She recently switched to the Sur-Fit Flange and Pouch System® (Squibb). Like so many people with a stoma, she has made some modifications. (Figure 11) She trims the 4" x 4"

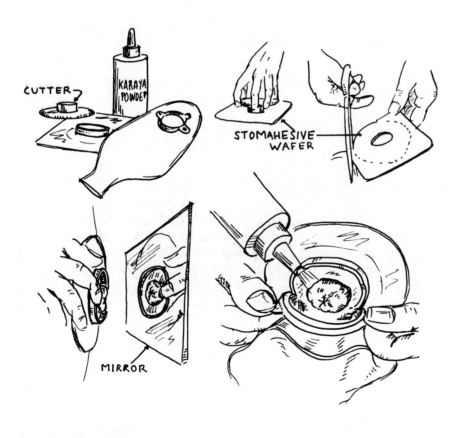

CUTTER

KARAYA POWDER

STOMAHESIVE WAFER

MIRROR

FIGURE 11   **SHELLY**

*square flange into a 3" circle. She cuts the inside diameter with a hole cutter to ¾";
her stoma measures ⅞". (She does not follow "the rules.") She uses her finger to
"stretch" the opening by pulling the cut edge of the Stomahesive toward the
plastic flange. She places this prepared face plate on her clean dry skin, checking
in the mirror to see that it is centered over the stoma. Then she "poofs" karaya
powder around the base of her stoma, even though the Stomahesive is snug up
against it. Then she snaps on the 10" opaque pouch.*

*She does not use a belt. When she's going swimming, skiing, etc., she rein-
forces the flange edges with pink plastic tape. Other times she leaves the tape off to
allow the skin to "rest." She prefers a plastic tail closure with rubber bands
(United) and carries extra rubber bands in the change purse of her wallet. Shelly
changes every fourth or fifth day in the winter but usually more frequently during
the summer. She snaps off the pouch to "poof" new karaya powder around the
base of the stoma each morning when she's dressing. Sometimes she adds some at
night too, particularly if she's had a day of watery stools.*

*Mike (See Figure 12) says that he's tough on his stuff so he uses reusable
equipment. He laughs and says that he's teased about being "old fashioned," but
then he winks, "I've had my ileostomy since I was a little kid." Mike is 5'9" tall
and weighs 175 pounds. The girl who sits next to him in home room describes him
as "a hunk."*

*His stoma is 1⅛" in diameter. He uses Marlen appliances—green neoprene
oval convex All Flexible® face plates and medium Odor-Ban® pouches with the
standard "O"-ring to secure the pouch to the face plate. If he's going backpacking
with his friends, he prefers the large pouch. He always uses a belt and reinforcing
tape strips.*

*Mike cleans his skin well with "whatever soap is handy," but he adds that the
oily "ladies' soaps are murder" because they leave a greasy film on the skin. He
uses a Colly-Seel® (Mason) that is pre-cut to the dimension of his face plate with a
1¼" stomal opening. (Byram Surgical) He places the Colly-Seel on his clean, dry
skin and presses firmly for about 30 seconds. Then he puts a Karaya Washer®
(Atlantic) with a 2" outside diameter and 1⅛" inside diameter around the stoma
like a collar. (Mike assembles the appliance as he is collecting up the items he
needs to make a change.) He laughs and says, "Only my mother could stretch that
pouch on the face plate after it was on me, and I don't want her messin' with my
'bod' any more. It works just as good this way." He uses the Marlen clamp
closure.*

*Mike adds, "I never go anywhere without my chewable bismuth subgallate
tablets to keep the odor down." He carries a supply in his pocket in a small plastic
snap-open change holder. Mike disassembles the appliance before washing it in
liquid detergent. After rinsing he hangs the parts to dry on hooks his father
installed on the inside of his bathroom cabinet door. He rotates three face plates*

and two or three pouches. He changes every Monday and Thursday night, "ex-cept during soccer season" when he changes every other day, "just to be sure."

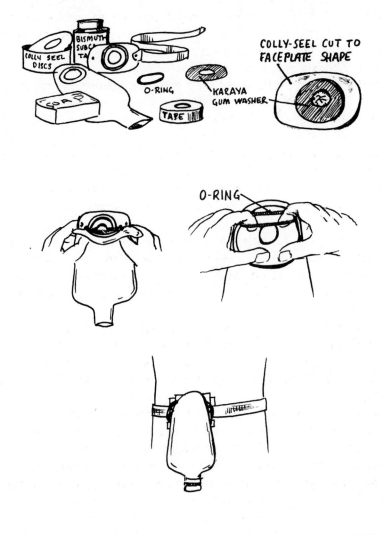

FIGURE 12   **MIKE**

Jeff and Linda use Karaya Seal Drainable Stoma Bags (Hollister); Rick prefers the Extra Ileo B pouch (Coloplast); and Don likes his "California system" that combines a karaya washer (Blanchard), a 3" round plastic face plate (Torbot), a saran pouch (Cryovac) and a rubber "O"-ring, with no belt but four strips of pink waterproof tape (Downs) (Figure 13).

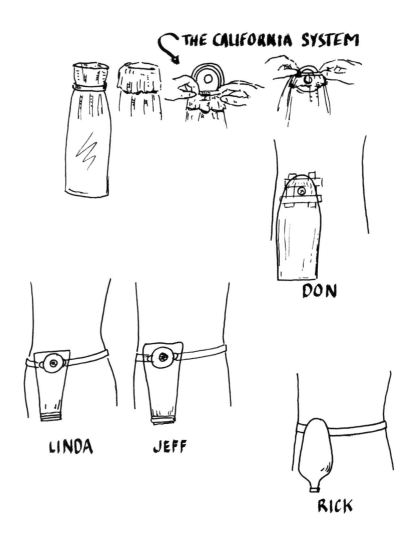

FIGURE 13   **ILEOSTOMIES**

There are dozens of methods and variations in ileostomy care. The best sources of guidance are an ET, a well-stocked surgical supplier, and chapter, regional or national meetings of the United Ostomy Association where appliances and accessories are displayed. When trying something new it is important to "give it a chance." It takes the body a little time to accommodate to new skin coverings and adhesives. Never make the mistake of deciding "it didn't work" after only one application, unless there really is an adverse skin reaction that causes immediate discomfort. The right combination of ease, economy, and comfort is essential in ileostomy care.

THE CONTINENT ILEOSTOMY

In 1969 Dr. N. G. Kock of Goteborg, Sweden, published the first report of his efforts to create an appliance-less ileostomy. Called an ileal pouch, ileal reservoir, a Kock pouch, or CONTINENT ILEOSTOMY, this operation creates an internal sac or reservoir made from the end of the small intestine. (Figure 14) The pouch is made with a valve created from the intestine itself and this valve prohibits the passage of stool and most gas. It is emptied regularly, every four to six hours after it has been in place for some time, by inserting a special catheter with large openings and draining off the ileal contents. If the stool gets too thick, a small amount of water can be inserted through the catheter to thin it out.

The Kock pouch is not advised for anyone with Crohn's disease, but it is an exciting new kind of ileostomy for patients with ulcerative colitis. There is a stoma; but because no appliance is required, it may be placed much lower on the abdomen. This permits the wearing of skimpier bathing suits and lower cut jeans. Now that the early complications associated with the Kock reservoir have been greatly reduced, many people with a conventional ileostomy are "trading it in" for a continent one. On the other hand, others feel that their present ileostomies aren't troublesome enough to warrant such elective surgery.

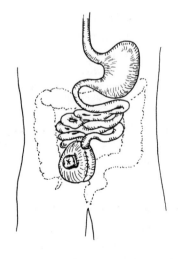

FIGURE 14   CONTINENT ILEOSTOMY

Dr. Irwin Galernt of Mount Sinai Hospital in New York believes that it is important for patients to be old enough to manage their continent ileostomies. He has concluded that their summer between the junior and senior year of high school or following graduation are about the right age. According to Dr. Galernt, it probably is not a good idea to perform a continent ileostomy on children under 16. For now, at least, a conventional ileostomy is the operation of choice for young people with inflammatory bowel disease.

By their own testimony, none would exchange their ileostomy for the symptoms that led to it.

Ileostomy Questions

- Does it show?

  Ileostomy appliances are not noticeable under most normal clothing. Some thin material and filmy garments permit a silhouette that would be recognized by a keen eye.

- Does it hurt?

  No, there is no pain associated with the stoma itself. There may be "phantom pain" where the rectum has been removed and the feeling of needing to have a bowel movement recurs. There may also be the abdominal discomfort common after surgery, and there may be a feeling of rectal fullness and discomfort when the rectum is left in place, but the stoma should not be a source of pain.

- How often must appliances be changed?

  Appliances generally must be changed more frequently on younger children than adults (often 2 or 3 times a week). Children are not as careful about emptying; they get dirtier at play and need more baths; and their small abdomens have less space to accommodate an appliance without interference from skin folds and creases.

- How old are children before they can change their own appliances?

  Of course this varies, but young children should be encouraged to participate. They can get their supplies out of the cabinet, hold a gauze pad or tissue, or help wash their skin. Six and seven-year-olds are about ready to assume full responsibility, so they can change or direct a change when they are at school or away from home. This does not mean that they don't continue to need gentle supervision and support and help with laundering reusable items. There is a fine line between nurturing independence and giving the children too much responsibility, but the sooner the children can be independent of their parents in ileostomy care, the more freedom they will be able to enjoy and the more opportunities they will have.

How Urostomies Are Constructed

UROSTOMY has become the catch-all term for the many methods of diverting urine away from the bladder to the outside of the body. Each has its own characteristics; in particular, some are more suitable for a short period of time and to a specific age group than others.

A NEPHROSTOMY (Figure 15) is an opening into the kidney (nephro-), and is located on the flank. A tube (which must be secured with tape) is inserted directly into the kidney, and in turn drains urine into a collection device. It is not advisable to put the tube into an ostomy appliance because urine collecting in the appliance would easily slosh back into the kidney, increasing the risk of infection. Sometimes the tubes are circular to insure that they will not be dislodged. Straight tubes, such as a Foley catheter or a mushroom-type, may also be used. Nephrostomies are usually a temporary solution to a problem.

Often urine leaks around nephrostomies and careful attention must be given to maintaining good skin. An increase in the amount of leakage, or leakage when it has not been present before, may indicate that the tube is clogged and needs to be irrigated gently or changed. Some urine may get by the tube and down through the urinary tract and out the urethra. Children with nephrostomy tubes generally are permitted to take tub baths as long as the water level is well below the tube site and the end of the tube is connected to a leg bag.

The advantage of nephrostomy drainage is that it is direct and easy to accomplish. There are several disadvantages: A foreign body in the kidney is a constant source of infection; and there is also the risk that the tube will become dislodged, requiring prompt replacement (in a matter of hours) before the tract closes. Emergency room physicians have shuddered when families on vacation have appeared with a child whose nephrostomy was not draining or had actually come out. Parents, especially mothers of active children with nephrostomy tubes deserve stars in their crowns and gold medals for their attentive care.

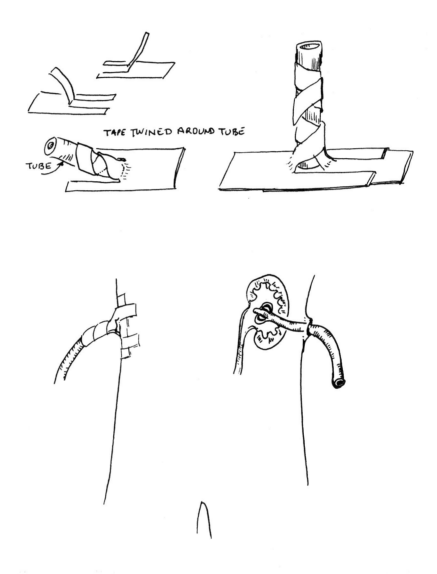

TAPE TWINED AROUND TUBE

TUBE

FIGURE 15 NEPHROSTOMY

Michael was just getting ready to start school when he required bilateral (both sides) nephrostomies. His mother (Mrs. F.) modified his underwear by removing the elastic from his Jockey shorts and sewing Velcro fasteners to undershirts and waistbands. He was much more comfortable without the elastic riding up against the tubes, and the shorts didn't fall down when they were attached to the shirt. Mrs. F. also made soft leg bands with Velcro closures to hold each leg bag. This eliminated the need for the uncomfortable rubber straps that come with leg bags. Her ingenuity made Michael's experience an easier one.

PYELOSTOMY means that the kidney pelvis is opened on the flank to permit rapid drainage from the kidney without the use of a tube. (Figure 16) Because of its location, it is extremely difficult in most cases to get an appliance to fit a pyelostomy, but it has been done. Generally, the easiest method of collecting urine is to wrap a diaper or thick padding around the waist.

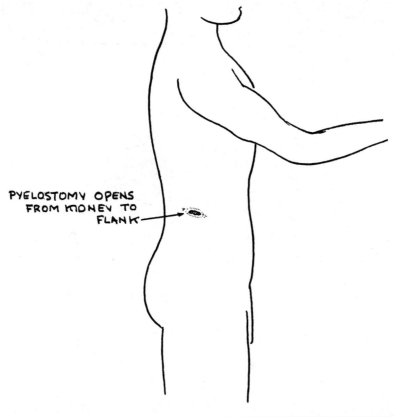

PYELOSTOMY OPENS FROM KIDNEY TO FLANK

FIGURE 16   **PYELOSTOMY**

There are times when the doctor will want the precise measurement of urinary output. The quality of the urine can be accurately assessed only if it is collected in some sort of a collection device, but a good idea of the quantity may be obtained by weighing the dry diaper or pads before putting them on and then again after they are saturated. Postage or diet scales are handy for this purpose. By recording the time and amount of fluid intake and the time and weight of diapers as they are changed, a reliable estimate of urinary function may be obtained.

Where it is possible for an ordinary stomal appliance to be used around a pyelostomy, it is important that the pouch be constructed with a non-return valve to prevent urine from going back into the kidney. With pyelostomies, as with nephrostomies, a tub bath is advisable only when the water level is well below the opening to the kidney. It is important to keep the skin clean by washing it each time the absorbent pads or appliances are changed. A protective film of Skin-Prep (United) will help prevent irritation.

URETEROSTOMIES may be constructed in a number of ways, depending upon the condition of the ureters, whether one or both will be brought to the skin, and the reason for diverting the urine (Figure 17, 18). Their location on the abdomen or on the flank, and the type of stoma that is constructed determine the kind of care they require.

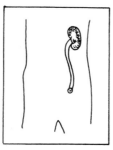

URETEROSTOMY

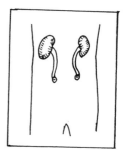

BILATERAL URETEROSTOMIES

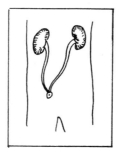

TRANSURETEROURETEROSTOMY

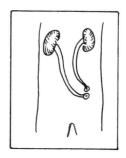

DOUBLE BARREL URETEROSTOMY

FIGURE 17 **URETEROSTOMIES**

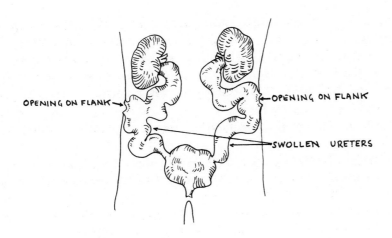

OPENING ON FLANK →

← OPENING ON FLANK

←SWOLLEN URETERS

FIGURE 18   LOOP URETEROSTOMY

On the abdomen a ureterostomy is usually no more difficult to manage then an ileal or colonic conduit stoma unless the stoma is flush with the skin or recessed. In children whose ureters have been swollen for a very long time, the stomal bud may look just like an intestinal conduit stoma. It is not uncommon, however, for ureters that are exposed on the abdomen to take on quite a different appearance. They may become pale pink and appear to be covered with a thin layer of skin.

All ureterostomies are more likely to stricture (become narrow) than intestinal stomas. This is a condition urologists will ask parents to watch for. Two common signs of stricture are (1) the progressive decrease in the size of the opening on the skin and (2) a decrease or change in the flow of urine. Should the normal continuous drip from the stoma become an intermittent "spurt" under pressure, this is a clear signal that the doctor should be notified.

Except in most seriously damaged ureters, after ureterostomies there is still peristaltic action in the ureters, carrying urine away from the kidney. This squeezing, milking action should prevent backflow into the stoma. Nevertheless, it still is advisable to use an appliance with an anti-reflux valve as an added measure of protection against urine going back into the system.

Most urologists allow their patients with ureterostomies to bathe with their appliances off. However, it is important that a pouch be worn in a swimming pool, lake or ocean.

When an abdominal or flank stoma permits the use of an appliance, stoma management will be very much like that of an ileal or colonic conduit stoma, described in a following section. When a loop ureterostomy or flank ureterostomy in an infant or small child makes application of an appliance impossible, the earlier description of the care of a pyelostomy will be more helpful.

If you are using disposable diapers, and using far more than you would be if your baby were urinating normally, discuss the situation with the social service department at the hospital. It may be possible, with some paper work and your doctor's authorization and prescription, to get the diapers at a reduced rate, or to have them covered by your private insurance or through a state or federal program of assistance.

A VESICOSTOMY is an opening from the bladder to the outside of the body. (Figure 19) A vesicostomy may be continent or incontinent. In a continent vesicostomy a catheter is inserted regulary to drain off the urine. In an incontinent ("regular" or "conventional") vesicostomy, urine flows continuously or at frequent intervals as urine collects in the bladder. The way in which the bladder is situated in the body dictates the location of a vesicostomy on the abdominal wall—about midway between the belly button and the pubic bone.

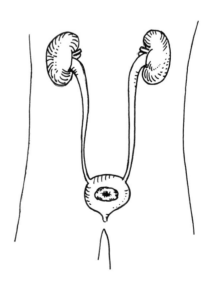

FIGURE 19 **VESICOSTOMY**

More often than not, a vesicostomy is very difficult to fit with an appliance, even before puberty. With the arrival of pubic hair, successful use of an appliance is made even more difficult. For this reason a vesicostomy is usually performed in early childhood, and planned as a short-term remedy.

Tanya (Figure 20) required a vesicostomy when she was two. At that time diapers were satisfactory, and there was no need to use an appliance. At seven it became important to find a way to keep her dry. Tanya's mother was able to use a Mini-Pouch® (United) with Skin-Bond Cement® (United) and reinforcing strips of Micropore® (3M) tape. She had to change it for Tanya every other day, but preferred this method because Tanya had been teased by some of her second grade classmates when she started school "still in diapers."

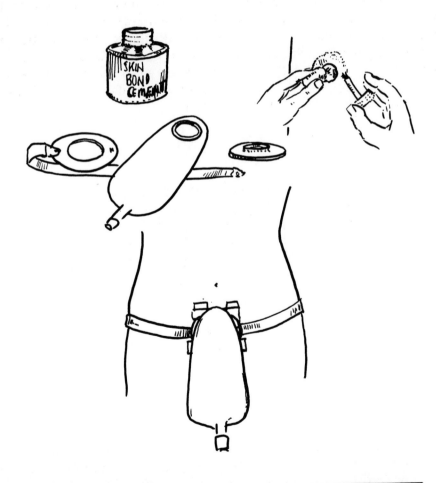

FIGURE 20   **TANYA**

The ILEAL or COLONIC CONDUIT are the two most common methods of diverting urine in children, when the bladder cannot be repaired or made to function properly, or when it must be removed entirely. In the early 1950s Dr. Eugene Bricker described the use of an ileal conduit operation for adults who needed to have their bladder removed for cancer. Urologists saw its usefulnes for children whose bladders did not function properly.

In the ileal conduit (Figure 21) a short piece of ileum, about four to six inches, is separated from the small intestine to be used as a pipe (conduit) for the urine. The ureters are put into one end, or into the side, and the other end is brought out on the abdomen. An appliance is worn at all times to collect the urine that drips continuously. Stoma location is extremely important, and the best site is selected well ahead of the surgery. For children in braces, on crutches, and in wheelchairs it is especially important that the orthotists and physical therapists be consulted, along with the orthopedic surgeon, to avoid conflicting with proposed corrective surgery or planned casting or bracing.

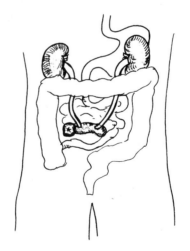

FIGURE 21   ILEAL CONDUIT

In the early days an ileal conduit was often called an "ileal bladder," which erroneously suggested that the piece of ileum substituted for a bladder and stored urine. It also was frequently referred to as an "ileostomy," because a part of the ileum was brought out on the abdomen.

Calling an ileal conduit an "ileostomy" has caused confusion, and has resulted in the purchase of appliances designed for feces instead of urine. An ileostomy appliance has a wide tail spout that is not suited for urinary drainage in the toilet and will not accommodate a drainage extension fitting at night. (Hollister, one of the leading manufacturers of ostomy appliances, probably was the originator of the term "urostomy," to minimize confusion when describing the kind of operation and the appliance necessary for it.)

In the late 1950s and 1960s many young people who did not have cancer, received ileal conduits because their bladders did not function properly; the operation was needed to achieve continence and eradicate infection. In those days there were only a few ETs to monitor stoma care. Nearly all appliances were reusable and few people knew how to clean them, or with what. Because no one realized the importance of remeasuring the appliance opening when the stomas' postoperative swelling disappeared, skin that was exposed to urine became encrusted, and actually caused strictures that resulted in urinary infection and kidney damage.

Urologists are concerned that although the results of an ileal conduit are generally gratifying and an improvement for the individual patient, some children still may develop kidney infections or stones, or experience renal damage, indicating perhaps a progression of existing disease. A search for further improvement in drainage continues.

In the past several years, some urologists and pediatric surgeons have elected to use a small piece of colon where ileum was used before (hence "colonic" conduit). The ureters may be put into this colonic conduit in such a way that urine, once in the conduit, does not flow back up into the kidneys. This is referred to as an anti-reflux procedure. (Figure 22)

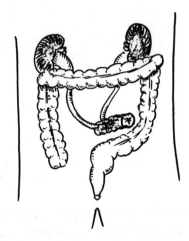

FIGURE 22   COLONIC CONDUIT

How They Are Managed

Besides careful application techniques to keep the appliance in place for several days without leakage or odor, a urostomy requires vigilant care to protect the kidneys. Observance of the following rules will prevent many stomal complications in children:

■ Keep urine dilute.

Drink plenty of clear liquids every day (four to six glasses).

■ Keep urine acid.

Drink no more than four ounces of citrus juice (orange or grapefruit) daily. Eat no more than one piece of citrus fruit per day. (Actually citric acid makes urine alkaline and reduces acidity).

Drink eight to twelve ounces (8–12 oz.) of cranberry juice daily. It takes a great deal of cranberry juice to acidify urine, but some is probably better than none!

Take recommended dosage of Vitamin C (ascorbic acid) if prescribed by the physician.

■ Protect skin from contact with urine.

The opening of the appliance face plate should be only ⅛″ larger than the base of the stoma.

■ Keep reusable appliances spotlessly clean.

Soak appliance in disinfectant available from major manufacturers according to their directions. (0.1% zephiran chloride has been shown to be an effective disinfectant also. It can be purchased without a prescription, but with a prescription it may be covered by insurance.) Rinse and hang to dry. Always rotate two or more appliances.

OR

Soak appliances in mixture of one part white vinegar to three (1:3) parts water for 10–15 minutes. Rinse thoroughly in cold water to eliminate odor. (Who wants to smell like a salad bowl?)

■ Keep urine away from the stoma.

Use appliances with a non-refluxing valve whenever possible.

Empty the appliance before it begins to bulge noticeably. This is a real challenge for busy children who forget or don't want to take the time away from play.

Use gravity drainage to a bedside receptacle for long naps or at night.

■ Keep accessories spotlessly clean.

Most elastic belts may be washed in the washing machine, but they will last longer if they are hung to dry instead of machine dried.

Night drainage receptacles and tubing should be cleansed daily with vinegar-water solution (1:3) or appliance disinfectant.*

■ Keep doctors' appointments.

Have urine specimen taken from the stoma by absolutely sterile technique at least twice yearly. NEVER ALLOW SAMPLES OF URINE FROM THE APPLIANCE TO BE USED FOR URINALYSIS OR CULTURE!

Children should have an X-ray of their new urinary system at least once a year. This may be an IVP (intravenous pyelogram) or a loop-o-gram. For an IVP, a solution that makes soft tissue visible on X-ray is injected through the vein. In a loop-o-gram, the liquid is inserted with a catheter through the stoma.

A final reminder: Dilute, uninfected urine does not smell bad.

Just as with ileostomy care, there are many appliances and varying methods of applying them. Monica, Renee, David, and Joe use four very different techniques.

Monica (Figure 23) is 16. She was born with spina bifida, and walks without crutches or braces. She was 15 when she had an ileal conduit.

Her stoma is 1⅜" in diameter. She uses an oval, convex grey Hypalon® face plate (United) with a 1¼" opening; a beige-colored pouch (Marlen); bead "O"-rings to secure the pouch to the face plate (United); Colly-Seel® (Mason); Skin-Prep Wipes® (United); Scanpor® tape; and a belt (United). She orders all her supplies from one distributor (Byram Surgical) where her Colly-Seels® are pre-cut to the size of her face plate and the size of her stoma. When she gets her supplies out to change her appliance, she cuts four or five strips of tape about three inches (3") long and hangs them on the counter. The Scanpor tape dispenser has a cutting edge. Then Monica puts the pouch on the face plate and secures it with the

---

*Recently diluted hydrogen peroxide has been recommended. Follow the advice of your urologist or ET.

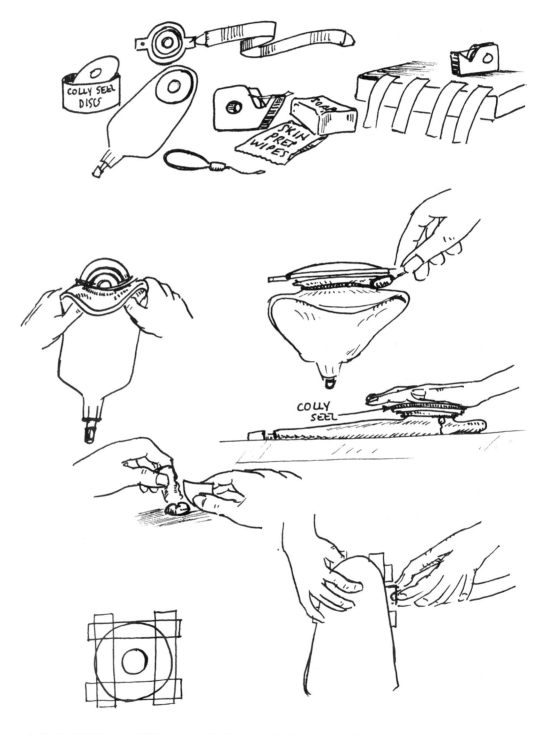

FIGURE   23   MONICA

bead "O"-ring. Next she places the Colly-Seel on the face plate and applies gentle pressure with her hand for about a minute.

On the days she changes, Monica likes to shower or bathe without an appliance. She washes the peristomal skin well with non-oily bath soap. When she uses bath oil in the tub, she is very careful to clean the skin around the stoma afterward to remove "the greasies." After blotting the skin dry with her bath towel she uses a Skin-Prep Wipe over the area that will be covered by the appliance and tape strips. She allows that to dry until shiny and slick. Then she rolls some toilet or facial tissue in a cylinder and holds it on the stoma to keep the urine from dribbling on the prepared skin. As soon as the Skin-Prep has dried, she places the appliance over her stoma and holds the face plate with one hand while attaching the belt with the other. Then she applies the strips of tape all around. In only 2½ months since surgery she has become a real "whiz" and takes it for granted that the appliance will not leak before it is changed every fifth day.

She smiles when she remembers how hard it seemed at first and how often the appliance leaked when she was learning. Thank goodness those memories are fading. She now is proud of her accomplishments and grateful not to be wet anymore, and especially grateful not to have to take medicine for the kidney infection that has been eliminated.

Renee (Figure 24) is a tall twelve-year-old. She has a very flat abdomen, a 1" protruding stoma, and a simple routine. She wears a Hi-Pockets Urinary Appliance® (Nu-Hope) with a 1⅛" opening, and a belt. She changes every third day. She uses Uni-Solve Adhesive Remover® (United) and tincture of benzoin (from a pharmacy or surgical supplier without prescription).

Prior to getting into the shower, Renee moistens a non-sterile gauze pad with Uni-Solve and wipes at the outer edge of the appliance face plate until it lifts easily away from the skin. She continues this motion until the appliance has been removed and then wipes any remaining adhesive from her skin with the other side of the gauze square. After her shower she dries the peristomal skin (the skin surrounding the stoma) well and applies tincture of benzoin with a Q-Tip® or the applicator that comes in some bottles of the benzoin (Bryam).

Benzoin is dry when it is tacky. While it is drying, Renee holds a tampon on the stoma to absorb the urine. (Her mother buys the cheapest brand in large quantities when they are on sale.) When the benzoin has dried, she peels the paper off the surface of the Hi-Pockets appliance and carefully, but quickly, centers it over the stoma and presses it firmly against her skin for 30–60 seconds. She attaches the belt and checks to make certain the outlet valve is tightly closed. She then discards the used appliance, tampon, and gauze pad in yellow scrap bags she keeps in the bathroom closet. Four other people use this lavatory and when she isn't tidy, they gripe and her mother nags!

At school and on field trips, Renee carries one Uni-Solve Wipe, one Skin-Prep Wipe (instead of benzoin) and one Hi-Pockets appliance. Should unexpected leak-

age occur, she can make a change with just those few supplies and feel secure until she gets home and can "do it right." She changes every third day.

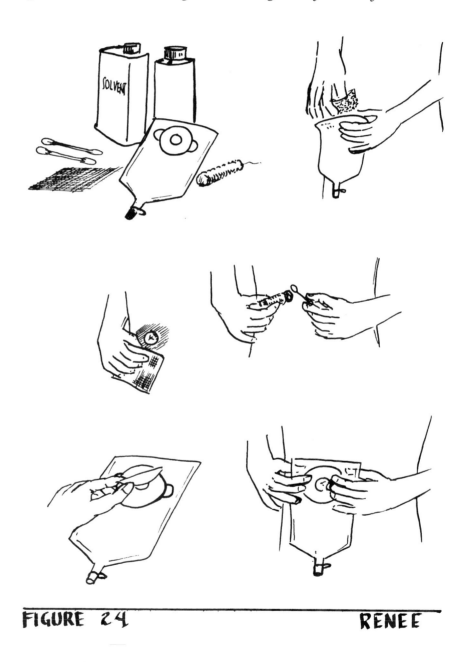

FIGURE 24   RENEE

David (Figure 25) is only four. His stoma is ¾" in diameter. His mother uses a Mini-Pouch (United) with adhesive discs and precut support strips that are made

for this appliance. The face plate opening and the adhesive disc are ⅞" in diameter. Mrs. L. (his mother) changes David's appliance every third morning except when leakage requires that it be done sooner.

Mrs. L. first assembles a couple of non-sterile gauze pads, Uni-Solve adhesive remover, a Skin-Prep Wipe, a clean latex appliance (face plate and pouch assembled), a belt and retainer ring, an adhesive disc, and two support strips. Then

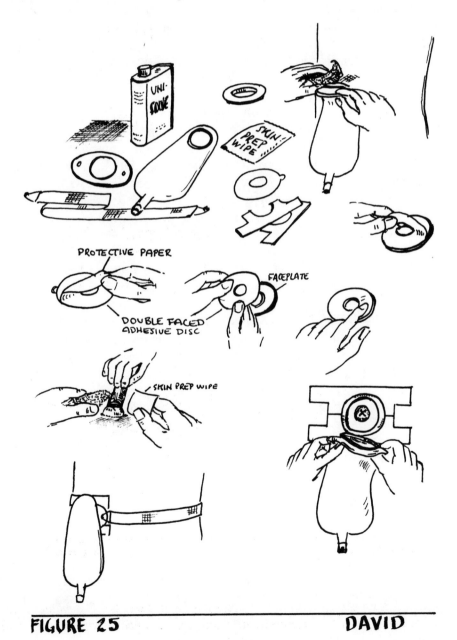

FIGURE 25   **DAVID**

she calls David and puts some Uni-Solve on a gauze pad and gently wipes between the face plate and the skin to loosen the adhesive bond so there is no discomfort in the removal process or irritation caused by peeling it off.

While David gets in the bathtub to play and wash, Mrs. L. peels the release paper off one side of the adhesive disc and places the sticky surface against the face plate. After she has rubbed around and around with her index finger to eliminate possible wrinkles in the adhesive, she removes the protection paper to expose the tacky surface that will go on David's skin. When he gets out of the bathtub, he wraps in a bath towel and heads for his bed where a waterproof pad is the signal for him to lie down. His job is to hold a rolled gauze square to prevent urine from leaking on the peristomal skin and then to hand his mother the support strips when she is ready for them.

She dries his skin thoroughly and applies Skin-Prep to the area that will be covered by the face plate and support strips. Occasionally there is burning if there are breaks in the skin. David yells and Mrs. L. blows and fans until the burning ceases. (When she notices reddened skin she warns him that there will be the burning for a moment.) Once the Skin-Prep is dry, Mrs. L. centers the appliance over the stoma. She was never happy trying to stretch the pouch over the face plate after it was on, so she uses the Mini-Pouch as if it were a one-piece appliance, even when she washes it. Then she places the adhesive support strips over the face plate edges and attaches the retainer ring and belt. While David is dressing himself, Mrs. L. puts the other appliance in to soak and puts things away.

Mr. L. is just as good at the procedure as Mrs. L. and takes charge whenever he has a day off during the week and on weekends. There are other people who can and do care for David: his grandmother, an uncle, and a 17-year-old babysitter who is proud of knowing how to change him when necessary. When David goes to the hospital, he can direct anyone, and loudly corrects the nurse or physician who strays from the regular routine!

Joe (Figure 26) is 18 and uses yet another system. He has a 1" circular stoma that protrudes at least ½" from his abdomen. He wears a regular size Coloplast Stoma Urine® (Bard Home Health), and E-Z Comfort Belt® (Parthenon) and uses a small Stomahesive wafer that he cuts from a larger square. He uses a cutter to make a 1" center hole in the Stomahesive. He uses scissors to cut the stoma opening in the Coloplast opening, just a little beyond the 1" marking guide. Then he cuts the 4" × 4" Stomahesive wafer into a circle, about 2¾" to 3" in diameter. He needs the Stomahesive because he has a troublesome scar from an earlier operation near the stoma and leakage occurs in that one place without the Stomahesive to fill the crevice.

After Joe showers, he dries his skin "pretty well," peels the protective paper from the Stomahesive, puts the wafer around his stoma, and presses it firmly, using a circular motion with his index finger. Then he peels the protective paper

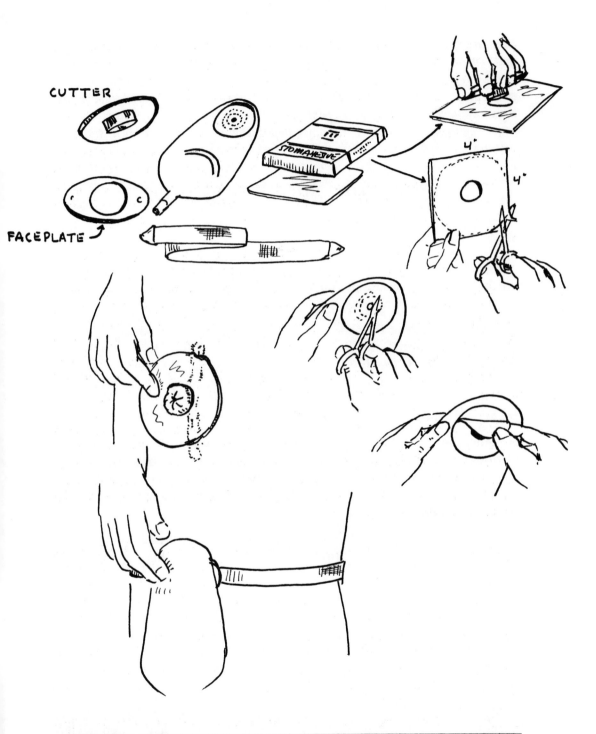

CUTTER

FACEPLATE

FIGURE 26   JOE

from the adhesive surface of the appliance and carefully places it over Stomahesive and skin. Again he uses his index finger to rub in a circular motion, from the base of the stoma outward, to promote a good seal. He slips a plastic belt retainer in place, attaches the belt, checks the outlet valve to be certain it's closed tightly, and discards the used appliance and paper pieces.

Joe changes every three to five days, depending on the weather and his athletic activities.

A WORD ABOUT STOMAHESIVE AND URINE

Stomahesive is a valuable skin barrier but it does melt rapidly when in contact with urine. There are several things to remember:

1. Some urine melts Stomahesive more rapidly than others. Whether this is because of the pH (acid-alkaline balance), medication, or infection is unclear.

2. The combination of some urine with Stomahesive produces a putrid odor that should not be confused with infection. By removing the appliance and smelling the urine that comes directly from the stoma a distinction can be made before becoming alarmed. Occasionally the odor may linger offensively in the bathroom even after the toilet has been flushed.

3. Stomahesive residue washes down into appliances and causes the inner surfaces to stick together. There is now a product on the market specifically to remove the tackiness; but unless it is absolutely necessary because of damaged skin, it is best not to use Stomahesive with a reusable appliance around a urostomy stoma.

A URETEROSIGMOIDOSTOMY should be mentioned here though it does not result in an abdominal or flank stoma. In this operation the ureters are implanted into the sigmoid colon and the rectum is used to store both stool and urine. (Figure 27) It is thought by some to be preferable to having an ostomy and an appliance; and when infection can be controlled and continence can be achieved, there are certainly definite advantages to eliminating an appliance. However, when children have a neurogenic bowel, when they have had rectal prolapse (a protruding out of the rectal mucosa through the anus), or when they have a weak anal sphincter that will not hold liquid stool, they cannot be considered for ureterosigmoidostomy. Ureterosigmoidostomy patients require life-long careful follow-up, checking for any changes in bowel habits or characteristics. Any sign of rectal bleeding calls for prompt evaluation by the physician.

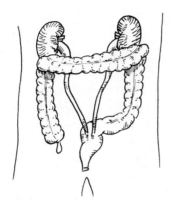

FIGURE 27   URETEROSIGMOIDOSTOMY

There is no operation that is guaranteed free of complications, but urostomies have, in the past, had too many. This is not intended to frighten you. It is intended to inform you—to explain why your urologist may think a urostomy ill-advised for your child even though many older children in the clinic have stomas; and to impress upon you the necessity of keeping appointments with your physician, and of being doggedly attentive to cleanliness in appliances and accessories.

There are urologists and ETs who are able to list a large number of young patients for whom a urostomy has meant freedom from repeated urinary tract infections and the embarrassment of wetness, and for whom stomal stenosis, stones, and other complications have not been a problem. The diligent care their parents have taken, or that they themselves have given their ostomy, most certainly has contributed to the long-term success of their operation.

In the 1960s parents were told that the ileal conduit surgery their children needed was "irreversible." In many books it is called "permanent urinary diversion" to distinguish it from a ureterostomy or vesicostomy that could be closed more easily. However, in recent years Dr. W. Hardy Hendren of the Massachusetts General Hospital and some of his colleagues in other parts of the country have successfully "undiverted" a number of their patients. For a selected group of children and young adults, undiversion may mean restoration of normal or near normal urination, the removal of their ostomy, and the elimination of appliances. Even when the bladder has not been used for ten, fifteen, or twenty years, it may enlarge to acceptable capacity in time, or it can be functionally enlarged, if necessary, by adding a piece of intestine.

Few parents are interested in any ostomy but their own child's, at least until after they have gotten this one down comfortably. You have probably skipped over some of the preceding pages that did not apply directly to your specific situation. But you may want to go back later and will then find it helpful to know a little something about all ostomies, to understand why some people manage one way and others do so differently.

A stoma and the necessity to wear an appliance means different things to different people. More importantly, and the reason this book was written for you, is that stomas have very different meanings at different ages and stages of development. At the time of your child's operation immediate events and needs may occupy your mind. It may be weeks or months later that you wonder how teenagers handle gym class or ten-year-olds cope with a slumber party.

The variety of information that will be important extends to much more than just what appliances and accessories you need. There is much more. Now we will move on to a broader spectrum—about children and parenting, and how an ostomy might affect growing up, and how parents can be most helpful along the way.

Notes

The Children

There is in every child at every stage a new miracle of vigorous unfolding, which constitutes a new hope and a new responsibility

ERIK ERIKSON

Watching children as they grow is more than just a fascinating experience reserved for parents and grandparents. It is also a science that has consumed the professional lives of pediatricians, language experts, behavioral scientists, and sociologists, among others. Isn't it amazing to think that some behaviors in childhood are universal—that at nearly the same age children in Alaska, Argentina, South Africa, and Moscow will be able to complete similar tasks? On the other hand, some behaviors are very much a part of the culture in which children live. There are the behaviors that can be linked to family traditions and expectations; and then there are those that cannot be traced at all, and are simply a facet of a child's personality.

Recognizing that children's personalities reflect their biological, psychological, and social experiences, it is reasonable to expect that unusual occurrences, such as repeated hospitalizations, operations with extended periods of inactivity, and alterations of anatomy and toileting methods, will affect the kind of people they grow up to be. Exactly *how* is the question. The quest to plot a course, to predict "how they'll turn out," has preoccupied parents and researchers alike.

All parents believe, and rightly so, that their children are unique. At the same time it is comforting to discover some things that are common to most children, that ". . . Everyone's children are negative at two," and that ". . . Everyone's kids make up tales."

The following review of child development is only detailed enough to help you recognize the most common traits of maturing, as well as the uncommon events that are likely to make a difference to children with an ostomy. We hope you will find comfort in knowing what is typical, and take counsel from learning what can be done when situations are exceptional.

Infancy

The first demonstration of social trust in the baby is the ease of his feeding, the depth of his sleep, the relaxation of his bowels

ERIK ERIKSON

The period called "infancy" generally includes the first eighteen months of life. In the last decade or two there has been increased interest in the first days and weeks of life. Well-known pediatricians such as Drs. T. Berry Brazelton of Harvard and Marshall Klaus and John Kennell of the Children's Hospital in Cleveland, have begun reporting important new findings that are changing the way infants are being cared for in delivery rooms, newborn nurseries, and neonatal intensive care units.

It is now recognized that newborn babies see and hear and are quite alert to their surroundings. Even more significant is their particular responsiveness to a high pitched female voice. Videotapes have captured newborns gazing at their mothers with fascination for a half hour or longer, and imitating someone sticking out a tongue. It has been discovered that infants synchronize their movements to the rhythm of the human voice. The love attachment that develops between mother and baby is the result of a bonding process that begins during the pregnancy, with the mother's fantasies and plans, and develops gradually, after delivery, in a process marked by touching, looking, cooing, cuddling, and caring for the infant.

Babies are able to express hunger and discomfort with their cry. The attention their signals receive sets the stage for their first impression of the world. According to a famous psychologist, Dr. Erik Erikson, babies' trust in themselves, others, and their environment has its roots in their feeding and toileting experiences. Where there is consistent response to their needs, and comfort associated with taking food, urination and stooling—without colic or pain—a sense of trust in self and surroundings develops. On the other hand, Dr. Erikson suggests that early experiences of insecurity, discomfort, and inattention to basic physical needs may be the source of mistrust and a pessimistic outlook on the world.

Parents note that babies appear to be in perpetual motion when they are awake. The first stage of life has been called the sensorimotor stage. Infants learn by moving. There is pleasure simply from bodily movement. They learn by touching, feeling, tasting, and mouthing. When babies see that their hand waved against an object suspended over the crib causes the object to move, they will repeat the motion over and over again. Their first impressions of themselves—their body image—begin with relief of hunger and other sensations that come from within the body. Then they begin to explore their bodies, looking at their hands, chewing on their toes, touching every reachable part.

At this stage there is no frame of reference for infants to believe that an ostomy is "bad" or "ugly." The ostomy is part of the body they discover. The pouch and its contents are usually pleasurable discoveries. The pouches are easy to grasp; they make a soft rustling noise; and the contents are new textures to experience!

There are many messages that parents and caregivers can give. If they indicate that the ostomy is disgusting or shameful, saying "No, poo-poo!" with an ugly face each time an infant's hand moves toward the abdomen, that is the image that will build for the child. Usually the best reaction is very little obvious attention. When the ostomy is uncovered for care, it is best treated matter-of-factly with confidence and approval. At other times, its fascinating qualities are best kept covered! (The best way to avoid a mess that is certain to follow infants' encounters with an ostomy pouch is to dress them in garments that snap around the neck and at the crotch, or that close in such a manner that they are difficult for the infant to get into.)

Another type of concern relates to the pace of development. Parents should be careful not to give their babies negative messages because they don't seem to be on the development schedule that is regarded as "normal." Under any circumstances some infants sit, walk, and say words earlier than others. And when children spend a great deal of time in the hospital, have general anesthesia, and generally do not feel well, they have added cause to be slow to sit, walk, and talk. That their activities are retarded at a particular times does not necessarily mean that *they* are "retarded." Should you notice these words used to describe your baby, perhaps in a chart, or overhear it used in conversation among physicians and nurses, do not jump to painful conclusions. Ask for clarification.

Parents often can help their children keep up or catch up by frequently stimulating them physically and socially. Frequent soft conversations and passive exercises or massage are effective means of stimulating sick infants.

Sometime between six and eight months of age babies learn to distinguish between their mothers and fathers, and all other men and women who do not belong to them. This helps to explain why a friendly outgoing baby, who flirted with everyone in the grocery store and the doctor's office, suddenly shrieks when an unfamiliar person approaches. This phenomenon is called "stranger anxiety," and it has particular meaning for infants who must be hospitalized. Someone estimated that babies will commonly see more than 100 unfamiliar faces within hours of their hospital admission.

Many hospitals try to limit the number of different people who come in contact with their patients at this age. In any event, it is less frightening to infants when a parent is with them during each new encounter. A mother's lap or father's comforting embrace will lessen the fear. Toward the end of the first year, this particular stage passes (although there may be reoccurrences later).

In the second half of the first year, however, another "anxiety" arises that affects how infants react when they are hospitalized. Intellectually, babies cannot comprehend that a ball that has rolled out of sight still exists. No amount of coaxing or encouragement will convince them. Similarly, when their mothers leave the room and are out of sight they, too, cease to exist. A frightening prospect for an infant. "Mommy will be right back," has no meaning at this stage of development. Tantrums or withdrawal are common (and healthy) forms of protest.

Hospitals have created increasingly lenient visiting and rooming-in privileges but parents cannot always spend as much time with their children as they would like to. During this vulnerable period "separation anxiety" makes hospitalizaton particularly difficult, for both infants and their mothers. This too tends to pass; as they gain mental maturity, children are able to cope better with their mothers' absence because they can comprehend that they will return.

When long hospitalizations are necessary, with prodding, peering, and poking into every bodily opening, parents and professionals need to work together to cope with the inevitable social alienation. If a new baby can't be held, being swaddled in a blanket may offer security. A cradle may provide a soothing motion to an agitated infant.

Skin care to prevent diaper rash is crucial to an infant's comfort and sense of well-being. In the absence of an appliance, skin around an exstrophied bladder or a new colostomy should be washed frequently and protected at all times with a skin barrier.

All too often, unfortunately, sick babies don't eat well. They have stomach upsets; and they spit up. Distraught mothers may become personally involved and feel rejected or insecure about their ability to care for their children. But you cannot stoke up babies like furnaces. The temptation to "build them up" for their operation by force feeding large portions of high-protein foods is likely only to make matters worse. The best thing you can do is to pay attention to the sound nutrition advice that is available, particularly from the dietician.

Great care should be taken to promote exploratory movement and activity, even when babies are confined to a crib. Colorful crib bumpers, mobiles, and play activities brought to the bedside are helpful. Restraints should be used only when they are absolutely necessary. Moving the crib to a more central location where there is more going on also may be stimulating.

It is all too normal for parents of seriously ill children to become immobilized by worry. But trying to focus on what can be done often helps. Learning about the infant's needs, finding out what is expected of you, and planning ways to compensate for limitations will get you going on the positive side, and contribute to your child's progress.

Georgie was a memorable baby boy, born with imperforate anus and one very badly damaged kidney. He was in the operating room having a colostomy and a ureterostomy on his first day of life. Before he arrived in the neonatal intensive care unit, the staff had been alerted to his "other problems"—unmarried teenage parents. But with seemingly nothing going for him, he somehow thrived.

Rather than become overwhelmed by the "hopelessness" of the situation, his young mother and father became actively involved and took excellent care of him. A grandmother and two aunts were also attentive and became experts in his care. Despite gloomy predictions, he made amazing physical, social, and intellectual progress. His family's love for him and their efficiency with his complicated medical requirements most certainly contributed as much to his surprisingly good health as advanced technology and surgical skill.

Just as there may be no substitute for a particular diagnostic test or antibiotic, there is no replacement for competent and affectionate parental care.

Toddlers

This stage . . . becomes decisive for the ration of love and hate, cooperation and willfulness, freedom of self-expression and its suppression. From a sense of self-control without loss of self-esteem comes a lasting sense of good will and pride . . .

ERIK ERIKSON

The tasks that must be accomplished at each stage of a child's development have been likened to stairsteps. Each must be handled successfully for the child to be ready to go on to the next ones. Even if they're taken two-at-a-time, it is still necessary to pass over all of them to get to the landing and the second floor. There are the physical feats, like crawling, running, and talking. There are also the intellectual tasks—as well as the EGO TASKS that have been described by Professor Erik Erikson.

As remarkable as the first eighteen months have been, they are no more so than the succeeding year and a half. Toddlers, from eighteen months to three years, take giant social and intellectual strides. It's as if they have finished defining WHAT they were and HOW they were in infancy. Now, with mobility, vocabulary and mental maturity, reinforced by their sense of trust in themselves and those who care for them, they are prepared to define their individuality. The central theme of toddlerhood is autonomy: "I am." "It's mine." "I will." "I won't."—the anthems of the two-year-olds.

The terribleness of the "terrible twos" can be actually a sign of success, as the toddlers detach themselves from their mothers, determined to gain control of their world. (Small comfort often for the frustrated mother at the end of an exasperating day!)

In spite of the fact that it seems to be constantly at cross purposes during this time, the mother-child relationship continues to be very important. Try as they do to test their limits of freedom, children of defiance in the morning will cling frantically to a departing mother in the afternoon. If one can be separate, one can also be abandoned.

Routine is important, probably because it signifies control. In many households supper is preceded by a bath and followed by a story. When the order is changed, toddlers may feel that they have lost control. Their rage and resistance indicates their need to regain it.

By the age of three there is no mistaking which sex they are. The barber or neighbor who call Jimmy "Sally" is swiftly and defiantly corrected by the toddler. Even in the unisex American culture of the '80s, there are expectations, messages, toys, games, and attitudes that influence children's ideas toward their sexual identity. But, remember, their understanding is limited. They usually can only name five or six body parts and have no idea of what goes on inside of their bodies.

Their external sex organs are all tied up with bowel and bladder functions. They explore their genitalia with their hands, and boys often seem to hold tight to a little penis in times of stress.*

When sex organs and sexuality are involved, the social and cultural significance may be greater than the biological and physical implications,

---

*An exception to this has been noted among some children whose genitalia are deformed and who are incontinent of urine. Two research assistants at New York hospital noted that toddlers born with exstrophy of the bladder did not manipulate their genitals during their bath or while sitting in their cribs unclothed with the same frequency as youngsters with normal genitalia. The researchers drew no conclusions as to cause and effect. Perhaps sensation was diminished or heightened as a result of surgical repair. Perhaps constant wetness played a part in their disinterest. Other studies of older children with organ system abnormalities, such as heart problems, have shown that the children draw pictures of themselves with fewer body parts and picture the affected organs as much larger than all others.

particularly during early childhood. It is important to toddlers with genital abnormalities that their maleness and femaleness be respected and reinforced in every way possible. This is crucial in the development of their self-concept and body image.

Toilet training is a key issue for parents and for children. "Good mothers" are supposed to have their children trained early. "Good boys and girls" are supposed to be out of diapers early. That's the way it is in most Western cultures. Consequently, one of the most effective means toddlers have of resisting authority and demonstrating their own superiority is to toilet at their will rather than someone else's.

Although their mental processes are maturing, three-year-olds frequently construct faulty cause and effect relationships when one event closely follows another. If Tommy hits Ingrid just before she leaves for a hospital admission, Tommy is likely to think he caused her sickness. When children take a tumble or spill their milk following their mother's scolding, you probably will hear, "See what you made me do!"

As vulnerable as toddlers are, there are many ways to help them develop a sense of autonomy and to nurture their self-esteem, even when they are sick or have a deformity. Play has been described as the work of childhood. Through play children learn about themselves and the world around them. During play toddlers are able to rehearse and "explain" to their dolls and toys what is happening to them.

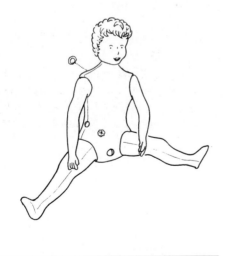

FIGURE 28   CHATTY CATHY

A popular educational toy has been made by drilling holes in a "Chatty Cathy" doll, where a nephrostomy and a urethra would be, and adding a realistic looking abdominal stoma. (Figure 28) By practicing with catheters, tubes, syringes (without needles), bandages, and appliances, toddlers can prepare for their own treatments. Teddy bears and similar childhood creatures may serve the same purpose.

Playing with their dolls often provides insight into their fears and feelings about their condition or the treatments they require. It is not unusual to hear toddlers scold and spank their playthings for "being sick because you were naughty," or being "naughty for being sick all the time." An excellent window to their fantasy.

Careful, truthful, and simple explanations are important. Toddlers may not fully understand what they are told, but they will be aware that a truthful explanation was offered. And a second explanation may well make the first more understandable.

There are many ways to let toddlers "take charge" of their ostomy care. They may be encouraged to "tell the nurse" or "tell Mommy" which things to put on the table, or to put them out themselves. They may hold gauze pads or a roll of tape, and otherwise actively participate.

The redness of their stoma is likely to be frightening to them. Remember, there are no nerve endings in the intestinal mucosa so there is no feeling. Gently coaxing them to "see for themselves" will help young children overcome this unnecessary fear.

Restraint and confinement are infuriating to toddlers. For this reason it is good to get everything prepared before calling them in for an appliance or diaper change. The less time they are told to "hold still" the better they will like it.

Their possessions are extremely important to them, and sharing is painful. When they have laid claim to certain items from the playroom toybox and another child or staff member seeks to take them away, reason and explanations of good manners are not likely to be soothing. When young children bring their own special toys and "lovies" to the hospital, it is very important that they be marked indelibly so they can be returned if they are misplaced.

When parents and hosptial staff can work together to establish a hospital routine similar to the home routine, this helps children retain their independence and feeling of personal control. Likewise, in the transition from hospital to home, young children need time to make their own adjustment. Toddlers may be irritable, tense, and restless when they are transferred from one set of familiar noises, smells, sights, and rituals to another. Limits must be set for them, even though this can be difficult for parents who feel their children have "suffered so much." Consistent discipline is important to every child's sense of security. It is particularly important in the inconsistent world of sickness and hospitals.

By the age of three most children have learned that certain parts of the body are supposed to be covered. Different families have different standards of modesty and conduct, but in any event, the ostomy question takes on special importance at this stage. Should doors be closed during ostomy care? Does this signify normal modesty associated with toileting or secrecy? Should the children be allowed to run around the house after their bath with just their ostomy pouch in place or should they be completely covered? Is it O.K. when the family is all alone but suddenly forbidden when guests are present? There is no prescription for correctness. The questions need to be raised and answered according to traditional family values and standards of behavior.

During this stage parents can help their toddlers formulate explanations about their ostomy when the appliance is being emptied or changed. A mother might repeat, "This is Kate's stoma. Dr. Nicholson made your stoma to help you get well. It's a part of your body now like your nose and your toes." It would not be unusual, sometime in the future, for her to hear Kate explaining to a playmate, "This is my stoma. Dr. Nicholson made it for me so I'd get well. It's a part of my body just like my toes and my nose." Beginning early to prepare children with ostomies to handle the curiosity and questions of their playmates is far better than worrying in silence.

Reasonable attention to clothing for toddlers with ostomies will add convenience and comfort. Playsuits with elastic across the back and straps over the shoulder usually are the most comfortable styles. (Figure 29) If you are buying panties and trousers with elastic encircling the waist or a stiff belt, first try them on your child. Make sure that the belt or elastic will not slip down and constantly undermine the adhesive seal of the appliance. It is O.K. to have a belt going across a stoma as long as it is not too tight and isn't positioned in a way that prevents urine or stool from flowing down into the appliance.

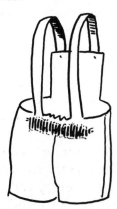

FIGURE 29

Mothers have offered the following suggestions for their toddlers:

■ If your child is in leg braces, open the inside leg seams of trousers and install Velcro closures to make dressing easier. (Figure 30)

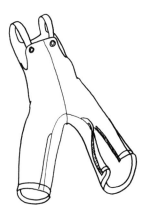

FIGURE 30

■ If your child has a urostomy that requires a bedside drainage tube at night, make a buttonhole in the leg of footed pajamas, around the ankle, for the tube to exit (warmth in the winter and less tangle). For summer pajamas, without feet, it helps to run the tubing down the pant leg. (Figure 31)

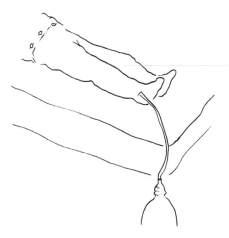

FIGURE 31

■ Cut a slit in jockey shorts and finish each edge.Put the pouch through the slit. This cuts down on annoying perspiration and eliminates the need for appliance covers. (Figure 32)

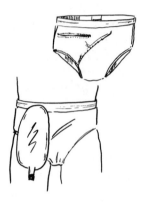

FIGURE 32

■ If your child has more than occasional problems with appliance leakage that can't be solved otherwise, use terry cloth training pants routinely for added absorbancy and comfort.

■ If your child has a urostomy, use a connector with a leg bag when you're travelling or visiting. You won't need to empty so often. (Figure 33)

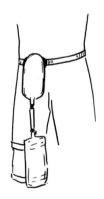

FIGURE 33

Children who are not able to establish a sense of autonomy are plagued by feelings of shame and self-doubt. Autonomy is essential for future self-esteem. It is a particular challenge for families of child ostomates, because of the extra supervision required by their illness, hospital rules and safety precautions, and parents' natural tendencies to overprotect children with disabilities. Creative strategies will be required.

Such strategies paid off for a little girl named Laura who required many hospitalizations during her young life. Her mother, Mrs. L., had worked hard to develop a cooperative relationship with the staff. With their help she was able to take over many of Laura's routine nursing requirements. She was responsible for maintaining the daily intake and output record for the chart. She was attentive but firm.

Laura had a special suitcase that contained a doll named Mandy, as well as catheters, bandaids, tongue blades, etc., collected along the way. Mandy's cloth body had been taped, pinned, and sutured in dozens of places. All remember Laura's mother asking her, "Would you like to eat the carrots or the meat first?" "Would you like to change your pajamas now or when we get back from X-ray?" "Shall we change Laura's or Mandy's dressing first?" Laura was in control whenever possible and wherever it was appropriate, but her mother patiently and carefully provided discipline and guidance.

When the children were resting and other mothers were studying the latest gift and clothing catalogs, Mrs. L. was always reading books about parenting. One day a young surgical resident complimented her choice of reading material and she said, "Doctor, when you are examining Laura and telling each other how pleased you are with your work, I want to be sure that I'm just as pleased with mine!"

Preschoolers

Initiative adds to autonomy the quality of undertaking, planning and "attacking a task for the sake of being active and on the move . . ."

ERIK ERIKSON

The years between three and six are marked by a series of grand accomplishments. Toddlers who have defined their separate selves are now ready to imagine and pretend what they can be.

With the drape of a tattered bath towel and the click of a safety pin it's Superman. With the smear of a red lipstick, a rummage sale hat, and a pair of wobbly high heels, it's a "mommy." Imitating grown-ups and heroes is an important part of the development of body image and self-concept. It is only logical that playing doctor and nurse would be so common, particularly among youngsters who have been hospitalized. More than one embarrassed mother has discovered her child checking a playmate's rectal temperature with an old crayon!

Preschoolers learn by experimentation and role playing. They can communicate with increasing fluency. Their attention span becomes longer and task completion and mastery takes on new importance. They begin to play well with other children. It is a helpful and cooperative age. It is not unusual for a five-year-old who is working on a model plane with a playmate to hardly look up when his mother comes into the playroom. Quite a change from the child who dreaded separation.

The important "ego task" during this stage is the development of a sense of initiative. It is necessary for children to have the opportunity to imagine projects, construct plans, and experience the joy of their accomplishments. The particular danger for children with ostomies is that well-meaning parents and caregivers want to shield them from bodily harm, and from failure or rejection by playmates. In so doing they may restrict normal and necessary participation.

At this time of life social horizons expand considerably—off they go, up the street and around the corner, to Grandmother's or Aunt Beth's. Parents of preschoolers with ostomies say they really begin to feel a crunch. They've invested so much time in their children's care and health. Wouldn't it be AWFUL if they injured themselves falling off a tricycle or jungle gym? "Children are so cruel," said one mother. "I just don't want Eric exposed to their teasing and curiosity." She had not thought how much worse it might be for Eric's development to be stifled by lack of contact with playmates.

Freudian psychologists and modern-day health professionals advise parents that sexual awareness is heightened during this period. Children enjoy the pleasurable feelings of masturbation. Their opposite sex parents and significant adults become important and the objects of admiration and love. It is not unusual for children to develop special feelings of affection for a nursery school teacher, a young adult, or a gentle nurse. What is important to children's emerging self-concepts is that these special attachments be respected and appreciated and NEVER rejected.

A blasé student nurse unwittingly rebuffed her little patient's expressions of love. His mother spoke to her in the hall and asked that she be more accepting. Though she was embarrassed, the student immediately responded. The next two weeks that she spent on the ward were happy ones for young Jeff. She would usually respond to his flirtations with, "You're special to me, too." And add a big hug. Good for anyone's ego.

The fantasy and magical thinking typical of this age group has special implications when surgery of the lower abdomen and perineal (between the legs) area are required. Children may believe that they will return from the operating room changed into the opposite sex. Boys may imagine they will be castrated, particularly if they have recently been scolded harshly for masturbating. It is important that preschoolers be reassured that they are not to blame for what is happening or about to happen to them.

Since they are still limited in their ability to understand parts of the body they can't see, demonstrations on models and mannequins and line drawings help them grasp explanations more quickly.

It is thought that band-aids are particularly soothing to four-year-olds for two reasons: they may fear that all their blood will run out unless the bleeding is stopped; and once covered, the hurt does not exist for them. Their thinking is often quite literal.

Examples of such childish perceptions abound:

A simple but mysterious procedure like a "G.I. Series" provoked panic in a child of four-and-a-half, who assumed it was a serious operation.

Five-year-old Tommy was heard telling his baby sister and some younger cousins, "When you get to be five, you'll get a stoma too."

More than one young mother with an ostomy has told how her five-and-a-half-year-old daughter asked, "When I'm a mommy, will I have an ostomy too?"

Some childish fantasies are humorous and harmless, but care must be taken—to preschoolers they can be frightening or demeaning, particularly in relation to their illness.

Ostomy care at this particular time becomes terribly important. The slightest odor of stool or urine will invite the taunts of other children who have so recently gained their own bowel and bladder control. It may be necessary for parents to put special emphasis on the importance of pouch emptying, to guard against leakage from over-filling.

There is a common reaction of mothers to nurses and ETs who encourage strict discipline in appliance care: "It's so hard when the children have been through so much." No one disagrees with how hard it is, but it will be harder still to cultivate self-worth in a smelly child who is scorned in the neighborhood.

What about trips away from home—with the nursery school to the bakery, or on a picnic with the Sunday school class? What about day care when mothers work? Explanations will be required. Even when an appliance is changed just before the outing, there are no guarantees against leakage. Parents of children with ostomies will have to plan more carefully and farther in advance. There are also several ways to compensate:

■ Some mothers are the perennial volunteer helpers. They do not miss a field trip. For many it is a delight, as well as a means of assurance. (For a few it is a resented chore or a way of keeping tabs on their child's activity at all times. These few do a disservice to their children.)

■ There usually will be one person in a day care facility who will be willing to take responsibility, after several training sessions. The initial reactions of fear usually disappear with understanding. One supervisor said, "I'll never forget the first time I saw a stoma. I thought surely it would get knocked off in the first hour and the kid would stop breathing." Now, she reports proudly that the appliances she puts on stay on longer than the ones put on by the child's mother.

■ A relative or neighbor may be willing to be "on call" when both parents work.

Social and educational opportunities are important to the development of a healthy body image and feelings of self-worth. Here are several suggestions:

1. Get a Medic Alert bracelet or neck disc. (See p. 135) (One mother had additional engraving added to the back: "Leaking appliance is a nuisance, not life threatening.")

2. Teach the child to give you detailed instructions by playing a game in which you "pretend like I don't know anything about your stoma." This prepares a child to instruct a stranger.

3. Prepare a one-page typewritten sheet of instructions, with the physician's telephone and other emergency numbers. Have the child carry one in a wallet at all times and keep a supply on hand for special events.

4. Send children away for the day in underpants that are attractive, but well-padded in case of leakage. NEVER at this age should undergarments resemble rubber pants or diapers.

When preschoolers must be admitted to the hospital, the routine and the required treatments may interfere with their toileting habits and their recently achieved independence. They are likely to be frantic at being called "a baby" or being made to sleep in a "baby crib" so soon after they've graduated to a regular bed at home. They may regress back to infantile behavior. The children will provide cues to their needs, and many can be met even in the hospital. Independence should be encouraged.

Though preschoolers are not quite ready to assume their ostomy care, there is much they can do. They can empty urinary appliances with relative ease if they have full use of their hands. Stool might be difficult to get out of an appliance and some assistance may be required. They can wash the skin around the ostomy, help during an appliance change by holding gauze or tissue to the stoma, arrange their medication for the day, and help tidy up. Even for children whose mobility is impaired, emphasis should be placed on what can be done, instead of what cannot be done.

It will not always be easy—to let the children climb a tree when you're afraid they'll injure their stoma; to spend a weekend at Grandmother's when they might soil the bedlinens; to go to the beach for the day with a friend without wondering how they'll handle changing clothes. In fact, each new invitation or opportunity may well create fresh worry and renewed temptation to say "no." But such temptations are usually in the best interest of anxious parents, not of growing children. Each new challenge they take in stride will fortify them for the next, and give them the confidence that promotes independence, initiative, and a positive regard for their capabilities.

Marcy was a five-year-old who had been encouraged to make the most of her potential. She wore two short leg braces and a urinary appliance. During one clinic visit a young medical student asked her what she could do. She began proudly reciting the litany of her accomplishments: "I can swim and ride horses and play the drums, and ride my trike faster than Nancy, and . . . [she paused to catch a breath and a fantasy] . . . do beautiful ballet and twenty-eleven cartwheels on the front lawn."

Middle Childhood

. . . this is socially a most decisive stage: since industry involves doing things beside and with others, a first sense of division of labor and of differential opportunity . . . develops at this time

ERIK ERIKSON

Mothers remember forever the feelings they experienced when their small children disappeared into a large yellow school bus for the first time or when they let go of a clammy little hand at the door of the first grade classroom. For mothers of children with ostomies, the memories may be all the more vivid.

The beginning of school often signals the end of a mother's extraordinary investment of time and energy in her child. Mrs. H. summed it up:

"Frankly, I wondered if he didn't need me any more if he'd still love me." Perhaps all mothers share this concern but with less intensity. The beginning of school for children with ostomies marks the real test of their mettle. They will have to answer questions about themselves, take care of an occasional appliance leak at a most inopportune time, and many will have to decide whether to participate in regular gym class or to request adaptive P.E. Entry into school and middle childhood heralds new independence, new adjustments, and new achievements.

Industriousness is the key to self-assurance, and the alternative to feelings of inferiority. Children will learn to read, write and calculate. They will be challenged to compete on friendly and not-so-friendly playing fields. Their social circle will continue to enlarge. Classmates and friends will become increasingly important and influential, and it will seem as if everything must be "checked out" with them, and measured against their standards.

Social, academic and physical accomplishments are necessary for status in the group. The easiest way in is to have a talent or skill that the gang admires. An underachiever may have to find an alternate route, such as adopting the role of the class clown to gain attention; at this age, there is no misery worse than being rejected or ignored. And children must earn their way into a group.

During middle childhood playmates tend to be of the same sex, and older role models and heroes of the same sex become significant in the development of body image and self-concept. A nine-year-old will cherish every moment she is allowed to spend with the college-age girl next door. She may be seen imitating her idol in the mirror. Seven-year-old boys usually have a club with "No girls allowed!" Often they take on the parts of popular television heroes.

Tall tales and minor shoplifting are not unusual. Most children remember being herded to the store manager to apologize and offer to pay for the piece of bubble gum or water pistol they couldn't resist. They may lie to avoid punishment. Parenting courses and books describe strategies of discipline that guard against backing youngsters into a corner where it becomes difficult NOT to lie.

Between school and play children seem to be away from the house during most of the daylight hours, but home is still a haven of safety and security—particularly when things are amiss outside.

Biological maturity accounts for increasing intellectual sophistication. At four and five years old children perceived a nurse as just that. She can't be a "mommy," "an aunt," or anyone's sister. But at seven the varied dimensions of a person or event can be understood. This makes it easier to explain diagnostic tests, hospital procedures and rules, and what will happen during a particular operation. Separations from family are more tolerable than they were earlier, but less so from friends, who will be missed terribly. A bundle of letters and drawings from classmates does wonders for hospitalized children's morale.

One of the most obvious characteristics of middle childhood is the importance of being just like everyone else. The type of shoes, the haircut, the lunchbox—and even its contents—must be the same as everyone else's! What, then, of the children with real anatomical differences? How do they make their way through middle childhood?

The following pages record some of their experiences. The anecdotes were chosen to highlight particular dilemmas and examples of how they were handled. Parents crave a portfolio of ready answers and standard solutions. It is never that easy. Good answers and solutions are often arrived at only after painstaking care—after the children's condition and personality, the social situation, and the school environment have been considered. Circumstances are different for children in Spencer, Indiana than they are in Paramus, New Jersey; even more, they are different for the very same child from year to year.

Three questions top the list of hundreds: Can children go to regular school? Where should they go to the bathroom? What happens if the appliance leaks?

What about school? Only a few years ago some schools did try to keep ostomate children out. Vicky's mother was told that Vicky would be "much happier" at a school for the orthopedically handicapped across town. Vicky does not have orthopedic handicaps! Tom's mother was encouraged to enroll him in the neighborhood school, but the teacher suggested that he not come on the first day so she could "prepare" his fourth grade classmates. Neither parent was pleased with these attitudes. Fortunately many children encounter no such difficulties.

A Federal law (PL 94–142), which was passed in 1975, guarantees public education in the least restrictive environment for all children. (See p. 142) For most children with an ostomy, even if they have multiple handicaps, this means that they CANNOT BE DENIED enrollment. But that does not eliminate the questions, and parents must be appreciative of the school's concerns and responsibilities. Some children with complicated conditions, and years of hospitalization with limited social stimulation, may need more than "regular" school can give.

At issue is a child's physical, academic, and social growth. The whole picture must be discussed between teachers, school administrators, the children and their parents. Sometimes physicians and social workers can be helpful. Free and open discussion will enhance the odds of reaching the best solution.

In addition to "Which school?" there may be a question of "Which class?" Some children who have been sick a great deal, who have had frequent and prolonged hospitalizations, or who have sensorimotor impairment, may have developmental lags, learning disabilities, or a variety of problems that call for tutoring, special aids, or assistance. Many parents welcome this; some resent it, insisting that their child is "perfectly normal."

Chris and his family had an unsettling experience. When they moved to a new school during the second grade, Chris took his perfect first grade report card with him when his mother wheeled him into Hawthorne School. The teachers and the principal were enchanted with Chris's quick smile and precocious manner. All were confident he would "do just fine," even though Hawthorne had never had a "special child" in a wheelchair before.

But Chris's smile soon faded and his enthusiasm for school vanished. He brought home papers with very poor marks. A quick conference revealed that Chris's academic skills were far below his social competencies. Apparently his previous teachers had let him slide since he was so appealing, and his parents had had no idea that he wasn't up to the work. But good communication helped the parents and teachers work effectively together to improve the situation. Two other children in the school required remedial help, so Chris joined them for reading, writing, and arithmetic. The remainder of the day he stayed with his class. His art talents and his "spiffy chair" gave him status in his regular classroom—status that he might have lost if he had tried unsuccessfully to compete academically.

The bathroom? There may have to be special provision for children with ostomies, to be able to empty their appliances before they get too full. When teachers understand WHY appliances don't necessarily fill on schedule, or regularly between reading and spelling, and WHY drinking sufficient fluids is important to the children's good health, they are generally cooperative. It then becomes important that children with special privileges do not abuse them!

Now, which bathroom? Often parents want to make this decision before consulting their child or the school. "I want Melissa to use the nurse's bathroom." In some schools the nurse's bathroom is inconvenient; in others it is inaccessible. In some situations use of the nurse's bathroom would be so conspicuous that it would be harder on the child than use of the general bathroom along with some simple explaining.

As a general rule, parents and children have found that, when the pupil restrooms have doors on the stalls, it is best for children to use the same restrooms their classmates use. Despite the fact that most ETs encourage females to sit when they empty their pouch and males to stand, many girls find it easier to remain standing. It is unusual to see a girl's feet going the wrong direction under the door, and such a sight may well raise questions—the girls who choose this convenience had best be prepared to explain!

What about leakage at school? It would be good to say it doesn't ever happen, but it does. A few students can count the times on one hand; others shudder to remember the numerous occasions. John and Serena are not the first, only, or last to tell of their horror when they accidentally dropped their appliance closure and watched it flush down the toilet.

Children should have a change of clothes, a spare appliance, and accessories at school, unless home is close enough (and the youngsters can get in). No matter how attentive and available parents are, it is unrealistic to expect them to be "on call" every day of the school year. Someone at school should be prepared to help a young child, and detailed instructions should be on file, updated every year. All children should have a plan worked out, so if they must change at school, they do not panic. Preparedness saves embarrassment.

And P.E.? Children with an ostomy usually are discouraged from participating in contact sports, but there are notable exceptions. One of the leaders in the United Ostomy Association's young adult activities made the cover of the Ostomy Quarterly in his hockey uniform. There have been swimming champs, soccer stars, and baseball heroes. And some football players, too.

Competition, participation, and athletic accomplishment are tickets to admission to the "in group" and important to the development of self-esteem. Encouraging early involvement in individual sports, with family support, will contribute to the self-confidence of children who are too small, too uncoordinated, or too frail to play team sports. (For those who can't participate in any vigorous physical activity, collections are sources of pride and status too—stamps, beer cans, hats, rocks, etc., are something to share and to be envied. Another alternative is learning to play a musical instrument.)

Sports participation can represent a fundamental challenge, which must be faced by families: Are they willing to take some risks, in order for their children to participate in the mainstream of society? Their physicians can help them assess the risks. Some schools require that parents of children with health problems sign a waiver that releases the school from liability during sports programs. It may also be necessary for families to get additional accident insurance.

The importance of sameness at this stage of development accounts for situations that, at other ages, would go unnoticed or seem unimportant. A few children have become the target of suspicion and ridicule when they were always ready for a fierce game of kickball in the neighborhood—but in the library during school P.E.

Showering after gym class has been, and continues to be, a problem for many children. It is high on the list of big problems for youngsters with an ostomy. Most absolutely refuse to strip down to their appliance in the locker room.

Ted had a P.E. teacher who would not bend the state ruling: No shower, no P.E. The ultimate solution was not ideal but it was a compromise that he could handle. Ted was able to get into P.E. class during the final period of school. Afterwards he used the coach's shower and explained to his classmates, "You wouldn't wanna see my body. It would scare you to death. I got shot up during the war." Ted said he had been using that line for other situations since the first grade and no one had ever asked questions; but his self-confidence would not be universal.

Research has shown that children generally are more tolerant of leg braces and crutches than they are of facial disfigurement and obesity. When forced to choose, boys have been less able to accept the idea of handicaps that interfered with physical activities than girls; and girls less able to accept handicaps that were cosmetic and interfered with social relations.

Whether the evidence comes from scientific research or casual observation on the playground, children with noticeable differences—from skinny legs, to freckles, to glasses, to obesity—are more likely to be ridiculed. Children with an ostomy rarely will escape teasing at some time during their school career. How much they are teased can depend on the cues and the behaviors they exhibit. A group of fourth and fifth graders with ostomies offered these suggestions:

- Play it straight. Tell the teachers and your friends that need to know.

- If the class has gotta be told, the kid should do the telling. It should never be a grown-up who tells someone's secret or something about 'em.

- Get a hobby and at least one sport, even if it's ping-pong or chess. Get good at them.

- Don't get fat. That's bad. If you're fat, go on a diet. If you're on steroids, that's the pits.

- Don't lie about your ostomy. (Ted was in this group. He insisted that his War Story was not a lie, just a good spoof!)

- Don't let your feelings be hurt when you hear "Oh, Yuk!" and "Ugh, Groo-oos!" from your classmates and "Oh, you poor little thing," from lady teachers.

- Keep clean so you don't smell, and don't use those deodorant drops that smell like public toilets.

- Even if you wish you didn't have it, an ostomy is nothin' to be ashamed of.

Children who have been sick for some time, leave school for surgery and return with an ostomy, may worry whether "people will still like me." During their convalescence is a good time to work on how they will handle explanations, etc. They won't face the pressure of participating in organized sports until they are well healed, so some of the easier decisions may be made first. The opportunity to talk to another youngster or an adult of the same sex who has had an ostomy can be wonderfully reassuring. Sometimes decisions are easier to make after hearing what others have done in similar situations.

The dress code of middle childhood is as rigidly enforced as in a military prep school. Even if children have to BE different, they don't want to LOOK different. For most youngsters with ostomies, clothes are not a problem. There are exceptions, and often ways to cope:

- Ginny is extremely small for her age and it is difficult to find anything but "little girl clothes" with sashes. Her mother (Mrs. R.) thought of having clothes custom made, but a seamstress was too expensive. Mrs. R. was able to swap services with a neighbor. The neighbor sews stylish clothes for Ginny and Mrs. R. babysits for her.

- Paula is in braces from her neck to her toes. She has a colostomy and empties her bladder by intermittent catheterization. She wears wonderful dresses every day because pants would be too hard to get in and out of for catheterization. Her friends call her a "cool dresser."

- Bruce complained that his ileostomy appliance pulls his skin when it begins to fill. His mother sews a pocket to the waistband inside his Levis and cords. He slips the pouch inside the pocket before he zips his trousers and buckles his belt. Extra support. (Figure 34)

- Ross is a paraplegic with curvature of the spine. Getting his appliance out of his trousers to empty it is troublesome. His mother modifies his pants by opening each side where the pockets are and making a Velcro closure across the waistband. Instead of a "drop seat," Ross has a "drop front"; but when it is closed the alteration is invisible. (Figure 35)

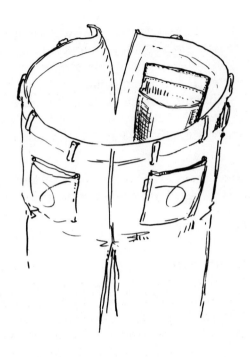

FIGURE 34

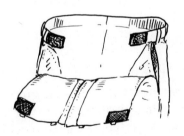

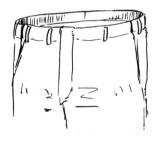

FIGURE 35

■ It's good to buy bathing suits early in the season while there's a large selection. Wide waistbands may help cover scars and tops of appliances. Bold prints and multicolor stripes or patterns conceal appliance silhouettes better than solid colors. An elastic brief worn underneath a swimsuit may provide a smoother look. (One visit to poolside at the annual meeting of the United Ostomy Association in August will convince any bystander that appliances need not be noticeable.)

Maintaining cleanliness is not easy for children generally, but it is critical for ostomates. Appliance hygiene is important for a number of reasons:

Clean reusable appliances last longer.

Clean appliances do not smell.

Clean reusable urostomy pouches minimize stomal irritation that leads to stenosis.

Clean dry skin around the stoma is more comfortable than irritated skin.

Clean dry skin around the stoma contributes to security against leakage and longer wearing time for the appliance.

Whatever measures are necessary must be taken to make certain that children with ostomies do not smell bad, that their rooms do not smell, and that they do not leave an offensive odor in the bathroom at home or in friends' homes.

As children grow, there are more opportunities for adventure—field trips, day camp, sleep-away camp, and slumber parties. To miss them is to miss important and memorable experiences of growing up. To participate means that some planning will be required and the children will have to take some "risks." John regaled a group when he described what he did with his urostomy's night drainage tube on an overnight camp out. (Figure 36)

There are special camps for children with various disabling conditions and health problems, but not for children with ostomies. That isn't all bad. Coping successfully with the experiences of a "regular" camp has proved to be the beginning of bigger plans, for travel, college, and eventual careers. Self-esteem is critical to the process of career choice and satisfaction. Some children with ostomies leave childhood with greater strengths because of successful adjustments they made and the knowledge that they had taken some hurdles courageously.

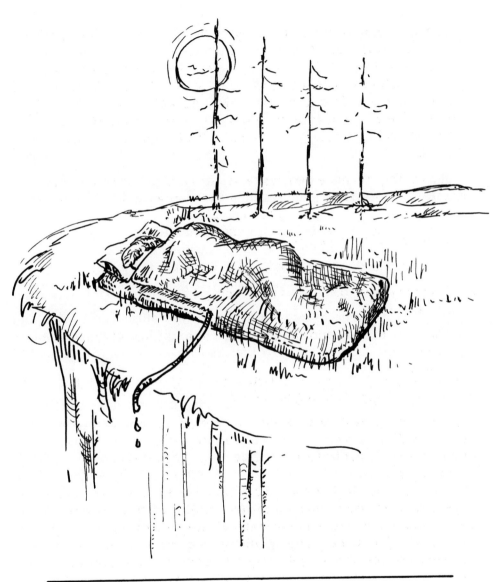

FIGURE 36

The story of Fred provides a good example. Born with spina bifida into a loving and determined family, he has been encouraged to make the most of his life. His father designed and modified an electric golf cart in which Fred, braced from his neck to his shoes, drives standing tall to elementary school down the street. He has a swimming pool in the backyard where friends often come to play—his limitations are less in the buoyancy of the water. He is learning early the good feelings of belonging and participating.

Adolescence

. . . adolescents have to refight many of the battles of earlier years, even though to do so they must artificially appoint perfectly well-meaning people to play the roles of adversaries; and they are ever ready to install lasting idols and ideals as guardians of a final identity

ERIK ERIKSON

"It seems like half the people are telling me to get lost while the other half are telling me to go find myself!"—the adolescent dilemma. Volumes have been written about adolescence, and the temptation to write another is nearly irresistible. Ostomies and adolescence can be explosive, but then, so can adolescence in combination with many events. And there are adolescents who say that being put to the test during their teens, and demonstrating their "stuff" has given life-long security and self-confidence.

Parents are frantic to know HOW ostomies affect adolescents and WHAT they can say and do to be most helpful. It is important first to review the developmental factors that come together in a crescendo during this period.

Adolescents are confronted with rapid physical change. They outgrow clothes and shoes at an expensive rate. Hair grows where it never did before; penises, hands, breasts, feet, shoulders, waistlines, and male voices change, it seems more rapidly or slowly than everyone else's. Tall or short, stocky or slender, "foxy" or plain, adolescents must accommodate to a changing body and come to terms with the physique that emerges.

Establishing a sexual identity and learning how to relate comfortably to the opposite sex can be time consuming. They are important first steps in the later search for a marriage partner and preparation for a family. But for now, one day it's dungarees and the next it's bare midriffs. Cosmetics, aftershave lotions, macho, and mystique are part of the teen culture. Memorable is the 9th grade football star who gathers his courage to coolly ask a girl to the dance. The next two weeks are spent in panic wondering, "What do I say after I've said 'hi'?" "Am I supposed to kiss her?" "What will happen when she finds out I don't know HOW to dance?"

A few close friends that form a clique become anchors when the rest of the world seems unable to understand. Hours are spent sharing secrets; asking for reassurance; dissecting, interpreting, and transmitting messages and sentiments between schoolmates and the guys and girls they "go with." A lot of life is spent on the telephone or at the after-school hangout.

A glaring and exasperating charcteristic of adolescence is the youngsters' near fanatical preoccupation with themselves. They posture in front of mirrors—preening, primping, and popping pimples. They are convinced that EVERYONE is looking at them. It's as if to say, "If I spend all day thinking about me, then everyone else must be too." A teenager dropped her purse in the center of a huge shopping mall during the height of the Christmas rush and a few keys and trinkets spilled out. "Oh-h," she squealed in pain, "Everybody was staring." The truth was, of course, that practically no one noticed.

In preparation for becoming adults, adolescents must define their own set of values, and sever finally the ties of dependency that bind them to parents and caretakers. It has been called the quest for identity, the primary task of adolescence.

Passage to maturity depends upon a clear conception of WHO and WHAT we are. Failure to establish a clear identity of self leaves adolescents in a state of role confusion, unclear about direction and potential. Thus adolescents may begin to take issue with family traditions, criticize or reject social standards, and ridicule parental practices. They are apt to relegate their 40-ish parents to pre-World War I vintage. ("Which war did you say that was?")

Parents become distressed when they mistake their children's philosophical experimentation and exploration for personal scorn. In fact, some psychologists express concern for adolescents who accept, without question, family rules and values. (They call such compliance "foreclosure.")

It is essential for teens to clarify their likes and dislikes, strengths and weaknesses, talents and aptitudes, as they have their first encounters with employment possibilities, and face choices about pre-professional education.

All adolescents benefit from opportunities to try out jobs, usually through summer employment on school work placement programs. Of course anyone with ostomy-related disabilities may require special vocational guidance. Often they need extra help and special consideration as they determine the kinds of jobs they want, and those for which they are qualified. It may be necessary to counsel the prospective employers.

New biological maturity brings new mental power—the ability to hypothesize, and to consider abstract problems and subjects. Not until now has the newly maturing adolescent been able to construct and discuss a variety of solutions to a given situation before selecting the best alternative. In fact, adolescents love to think about the hypothetical, the remote, and the future. It's as if they were exercising their new intellectual muscles with mental gymnastics. Some achieve this maturity earlier than others. Some have had encouragement and practice around their dinner table and in classrooms.

For some adolescents with severe health problems and disabilities, the new insight may lead to depression, as they realistically project, perhaps for the first time, what their limitations will be.

Not only is it important to the adolescent that certain biological and psychological events occur, but it is important that they occur"on time." An assembly of 14-year-olds is an amazing assortment of immature, mature, and in-between figures and personalities. Teenage boys are mortified, and their self-confidence suffers, when they are the smallest and least muscular in their class. They suffer if they cannot hold their own in athletics. Girls, on the other hand, may be shunned by their clique (at the same time they receive sudden masculine attention), if they are the first to become buxom or curvaceous.

In short, adolescence is generally a time of turmoil. Many consider it a war zone—a time and place in life marked by open rebellion and negativism. In fact, the teenagers in question may be demonstrating nothing more than reasonable physical and psychological growing pains.

What of adolescents with ostomies? Generalizations are always dangerous, but with one group a few generalizations can be made. They are the teens who have suffered with inflammatory bowel disease, whose social lives were ruined by fatigue, anemia, unrelenting bowel movements, explosive diarrhea, abdominal cramps, and malnutrition. Some will welcome the prospect of an ileostomy as a chance to participate in life again. Others will go dejectedly to surgery with a feeling of failure that they couldn't control their disease. But *all* will rejoice in their own well-being within months of their operation.

During the summer Youth Rally for young people with ostomies, three teenagers expressed particular concern about parents who did not want to consent to surgery for their children when they were too young to decide for themselves. They felt that their own ileostomies had been delayed for too long and that they had unnecessarily lost important years of high school fun. They were eager for opportunities to reassure worried parents and scared young people.

Several teens at the rally who had been incontinent of urine because of bladder exstrophy and spina bifida had had to "fight for" their urinary diversion. They were grateful for the freedom from pads, odor, and fear of embarrassment. One wrote an open letter on the subject for the United Ostomy Association's Philadelphia chapter newsletter. It is perhaps significant that all these adolescents had a number of friends who know of their original problem and all about their ostomy. Their acceptance and enthusiasm for their ostomies was impressive, as their frankness was educational.

For other youngsters at the meeting it had not been quite as simple as getting rid of a bad disease and getting back into the swing of things. For them, being small, sickly, and overly protected by nervous parents had been crushing to their body image and self-esteem. Their stooped postures, eyes to the floor, and unkempt appearance conveyed a clear message: "I don't feel good about myself."

It is easy to blame the ostomy. It is an obvious source of depression. But, in truth, there probably have been numerous factors that contributed.

What can be done to help? Someone always needs to listen carefully. Professional help probably is indicated, especially if a professional is available who is very familiar with ostomies and understands the few real limitations that a stoma and appliance impose. Family counseling would also be helpful, to demonstrate support of the hurting teens as well as to provide help for those who are affected by their unhappiness. The feeling of day-to-day support for the smaller problems can be especially important.*

Some public high schools, teen clubs, and community centers have courses specifically designed to help adolescents develop interpersonal and decision-making skills. If your child is one who appears to need such an opportunity, start looking now. Do not just gaze the other way and hope that tincture of time will heal the wounds.

And finally, along with outside support, there is no substitute for the family who cares and parents who provide optimism that their children will succeed.

Occasional anger aimed at the ostomy is common: "I hate it!" "I'd rather be dead than have this thing!" "How could you let them do this to me?" The response is often, "I'm sorry; we'll make it up to you somehow." A car, fewer household chores, more allowance, no curfew, no rules. This, of course, is folly.

Anyone has a right to be angry about having an ostomy, unless the anger becomes a harmful preoccupation. Often other feelings such as embarrassment or inadequacy are at the root of the problem, translated into anger.

---

*Stanley Coopersmith, who has researched and written *The Antecedents of Self-Esteem,* has concluded that recurrent problems are more likely to damage self-esteem than one or two severe or dramatic events.

Most of us are taught that it's uncivilized to be angry and that negative feelings should be suppressed. But by expressing our negative feelings we often defuse them.

As hard as it is to do, parents should try to listen attentively to their angry adolescents without taking blame, and they must resist the urges either to buy off, or to minimize the teen's reactions. When teenagers are hating their pimples, their red hair, or their beak nose, does anyone produce a set of keys or an increase in spending money?

School attendance often suffers, because adolescent ostomates dread the hassle and embarrassment of being behind in academics, or being shunned or simply unnoticed by their classmates. Many teens have dropped out of school in preference to repeating a grade or getting a tutor. Parents wanting to spare their children from such unhappiness often excuse their absences. They can be doing their children a real disservice.

Of course, high school is more than academics. It is a total personal training ground. Nineteen-year-old high school dropouts, with no vocational or social skills, and the added financial burden of ostomy management don't have much going for them.

Real questions arise about sexual potency, fertility, menstruation, and childbirth. Some youngsters are comfortable enough with their parents to ask them. Some wait until a physician or an ET invites such conversations. Others just wish they knew where to go or whom to ask.

Males who have had an ileostomy for non-cancerous diseases, such as inflammatory bowel disease, should be potent and fertile. (Potency refers to penile erection; fertility refers to reproductive capacity.) Occasionally there is nerve damage associated with the removal of the rectum that interferes with erection. When a young male complains of impotency, it is important to determine whether the cause is psychological or physiological. Hardening of the penis during sleep or on awakening in the morning with a full bladder are indications that the capability for erection is present.

It is not uncommon, according to a preliminary report given in 1980 by Dr. Hulten Lief of Goteborg, Sweden, for females who have undergone ileostomy for inflammatory bowel disease to experience some discomfort with intercourse, as a result of scarring associated with removal of the rectum. This condition is sometimes referred to as "frozen pelvis." At the same time, many young women with ileostomies have conceived and delivered healthy babies vaginally. The enlarging abdomen usually requires several appliance adaptations as its contour changes.

In males and females who require urinary diversion for non-cancerous conditions, it is not usually the urostomy but the original problem that determines sexual function.

For males who were born with posterior urethral valves, and who had an operation to open the bladder neck, infertility may occur. Infertility results when the bladder neck does not close properly during ejaculation and the sperm goes into the bladder instead of through the urethra and out the tip of the penis. Theoretically, when such a problem exists, it is possible to spin the urine that is voided after intercourse to retrieve the sperm. A urologist is the best source of guidance for this condition. Males born with exstrophy of the bladder may have a short stubby penis that is not adequate to penetrate a female vagina. Even when they are able to have intercourse, few have been fertile.

Females born with exstrophy of the bladder usually require vaginal repair before they are able to have intercourse with comfort. Some have conceived and borne children. Dr. John Lattimer and Michael Macfarlane reported on a number of females who had experienced prolapse of the uterus associated with pregnancy and childbirth. This, of course, would be a distressing complication.

For both males and females born with spina bifida, the degree of neural involvement will dictate the sexual adequacy and satisfaction they achieve. What is crucial for these and all young people is that their sexual conerns and needs be recognized. It is unthinkable that loving parents or health professionals would assume that "they've not interested in sex" or "no one would be interested in a sexual relationship with them." Unfortunately, there have been such misconceptions. Sexual energy, and questioning, is a part of every person. If anything, it is certain that adolescents with ostomies have all the same sexual concerns that average teens have, plus many more. They need a place to discuss them and people who can answer their questions.

It is not unusual for menstruation to commence late in adolescent girls who are small for their age or generally late to mature. Sometimes their periods are terribly irregular. Girls deserve to know and need to know whether their menstrual cycles are "normal," or whether they are affected by their disease or birth defect.

There are not a great number of gynecologists who have specialized in caring for girls with ostomies and associated conditions. It is helpful to consult someone who has had a fair amount of experience with these particular problems. Many young mothers, who were once hopeful young women with ostomies, were told that they "couldn't get pregnant" or "shouldn't have a baby" by well-meaning physicians who were taught this way in medical school.

When sexuality is discussed, so often people forget that there is more to it than "having sex." Sexuality includes attitudes toward our maleness and femaleness and relationships with the opposite sex.

What do young people with ostomies say to someone with whom they want to become intimately involved, physically and emotionally? How do they explain? For nearly every teen with an ostomy there is a story worth telling. Some are downright funny; others are sad and worrisome. Boys and girls report few rejections, some surprises, and many "Oh, that's all?"s from their explanations.

Generally the tone and manner in which the ostomy is described sets the stage for the reaction it gets. The best T-shirt at a recent United Ostomy Association conference was worn by a handsome teenager. It boasted, "I may not be perfect, but parts of me are excellent." The sad stories come from the adolescents who believe their ostomy makes their whole person inferior and who, for that reason, have not tried to date for fear of having to explain.

Sexual promiscuity is equal cause for concern. Boys and girls who are unwilling or unable to establish lasting relationships with a member of the opposite sex or to make an emotional investment in another person are showing that they need help. Many parents and health professionals have assumed that adolescents would be too inhibited by their ostomy to engage in frequent, casual sexual relations with numbers of partners. Not so!

They can be promiscuous for a number of reasons. They may be seeking reassurance and fresh new testimony that they are desirable even though they have a stoma. They may think badly of themselves and feel that they don't deserve respect—respect for their person or their body. They may believe they should sample a number of reactions to their ostomy in intimate situations before they can be sure they won't be rejected, or until they have been rejected as they expect to be.

No matter what the explanations, such behavior is physically and psychologically unhealthy. When people are secure in the knowledge that they are lovable and that they have something to contribute, they will not need to seek approval and reassurance from casual sexual encounters.

Acne is a less emotional subject than sex, but it is equally important if it causes daily embarrassment. A face covered by blemishes may be average teen skin or it may be associated with general health problems. Adolescents don't need any more physical imperfections than are absolutely necessary. Consult a dermatologist early.

Adolescents need privacy. They need it at home and they certainly need it in the hospital.

Charlene's mother told of finally getting up the nerve to "put her foot down" at the hospital when Charlene was thirteen. "The residents and interns came around and examined her without regard for her modesty and she hated it." "Finally, I blew my stack," she fumed. "Now only her surgeon examines her, and then it's in the treatment room and he's more careful to drape the parts he's not examining. I think he just forgot that she had grown up."

You may need to serve as your child's advocate when cherished privacy is on the line.

A word about drugs and alcohol. Drug use and abuse during adolescence is a worry for all parents. It should be a particular concern for parents of children with ostomies. When adolescents are not leaders in sports, academics, or the school's student activities, they are likely to look for a crowd where they will be popular. Often the group on the fringes is the group that gets by on alcohol and drugs. Furthermore, many teens with ostomies have had ready access to prescribed drugs like Valium, codeine, and Lomotil during years of illness.

The most effective hedge against alcohol and drug use is a positive self-esteem, talents that are admired by the leaders, and by children who are in tune with their families. A group of high school juniors told a class of adult educators that drug education in high school is too late. "It's in elementary school and junior hi, when you want to belong so bad and you're scared you won't, that the pressure is really on. In high school you either do or you don't because you're beginning to know who you are."

In a chapter for parents of adolescents with ostomies, any advice on clothing, appliance techniques, and hygiene would be close to worthless. Ever try telling adolescents what to wear, when to shower, or how to perform a task? They seem to be most responsive to anybody and everybody but parents?

This is why contacts with the United Ostomy Association can be so valuable. If the ostomy group in your community is too old to be appealing to an adolescent, at least a subscription to the *Ostomy Quarterly* will provide some reading material that might strike a responsive chord. Ask your child's surgeon where you might find someone of the same age, or a young adult with an ostomy who would be an effective role model. There is nothing like the good example of another ostomate to make a lasting impression.

There are dozens of other adolescent-related topics that could be (and should) be discussed—but not in an ostomy book. They should be talked about in living rooms, clinics, bedrooms, and at kitchen tables and on picnics—wherever adolescent ostomates and their parents, friends, and caregivers get together. Good communication is an important part of problem solving and goal setting. Bev, Mark, Matthew, Rich, John, Kevin and Paula are teen idols to many younger children with ostomies.

They have been leaders in the United Ostomy Association's youth activities; but, then, they have been leaders everywhere they have been. They have mastered situations that most of their friends could never even imagine, and they feel good about themselves for having done it.

Notes

Families Who Care

Children can learn to live with a disability. But they cannot live well without the conviction that their parents find them utterly lovable

BRUNO BETTLEHEIM

It is futile to discuss families as a unit without looking first at members individually. Then one can examine interactions and relationships—between parents, between parents and children, between children and children, and so on.

It becomes evident that each member adds a special fibre, and together, with time and events, they weave the distinctive fabric of family. When one child is delivered with a birth defect, or becomes ill in the process of growing up, the texture is forever altered. The family may grow stronger and closer; or it may become a chaotic battleground of conflicting and smoldering emotions.

It is relatively easy to write a book that describes specific skills needed to care for ostomies in childhood. But it is impossible to write a how-to manual on how to bring up children, with or without ostomies. K. C. Cole, author of *What Only A Mother Can Tell You About Having A Baby*, says it well:

How-to does not help us learn how to accept, how to improvise, how to roll with the punches, go with the flow. It presumes a life that runs on time, without hesitation, with no time out for late planes, broken hearts, lost jobs, sudden illnesses, unsightly blemishes or unexpected guests. So it can't help us cope with imagination and humor.

Parents of children with birth defects and serious illnesses quickly learn that, indeed, they need extraordinary amounts of imagination and humor, and also generous allotments of support from health professionals, family, and friends. What parents and brothers and sisters often find to be most helpful is a chance to see and hear what others have experienced in similar situations. This allows them to use some of the good ideas, improve on the not-so-good ones, and discard what is not right. How, then, have others coped?

Mothers

Mothers, it has long been assumed, are fully endowed at delivery with a plentiful supply of maternal instinct and love for their newborns. As was mentioned earlier, recent studies have demonstrated that, in fact, the bond between mother and baby is a process that begins before birth and follows a pattern after the baby is born. Knowing this makes it easier for some mothers to admit they "felt nothing" for their baby during the first visit.

Mothers of children with congenital deformities tend to experience a variety of rapidly changing emotions: rage, bitterness, bewilderment, anger, guilt, despair, confusion, and a kaleidoscope of all of them plus more. Mothers sometimes are "protected" from the information, and learn from whispers of the staff in the hallways, or deduce that something is wrong when their babies are not brought in for feeding. Mothers who are awake and participating in their children's birth get the news and feel the shock of the delivery room staff immediately. And then the baby is whisked away for treatment, sometimes to a distant hospital—even in another city—along with the father. Loneliness and overwhelming grief are likely to follow.

Even when the babies look pretty well at birth, several days of diagnostic tests, monitoring electrodes, IVs and nasogastric tubes are not flattering. Sometimes it creates a very frightening image. Some mothers have been able to admit frankly, "I just couldn't love him. He was so ugly." Others have said, "I prayed she would die. It was so awful to see her suffer."

The words of BAD mothers? Certainly not. They were expressions of feelings that accompany an event that didn't turn out anything like it was expected to; and that produced a baby that did not fit everyone's image of what all babies are supposed to look like—the ones in Huggies diapers on soft plush carpeting, and on Gerber's labels.

There are countless ways of being when you've had a baby with a birth defect—including being brave, being efficient, being wiped out, and being optimistic. The important thing to realize is that the way you are being is not ugly or wrong—until it does harm to others, unnecessarily causes you personal discomfort, or prevents you from beginning to deal realistically with the situation.

Some mothers effectively deny their children's problems. They seem to "tune out" all the bad news. They go about caring for their children and making plans with them as if they were perfectly well. For them, denial may serve as a valuable temporary buffer. It may give the day or week, or even months, of respite necessary to muster the strength to sort out feelings and values, regroup, and move ahead.

There are mothers who begin note taking, record keeping and researching nearly immediately. Within the week they have learned anatomy, physiology, blood chemistries, and all the hospital slang and jargon. For them an intellectual and scientific approach is more comfortable and less draining than an emotional investment.

There are also the inconsolable mothers. They conform better to the expectations that hospital personnel have. With every tear and long sleep to blot out reality there is evidence that they are "responding appropriately."

Of course, there is no RIGHT WAY to feel, no CORRECT WAY to behave in such times. Each of us does the best we can with whatever resources we have.

When mothers of children with ostomies gather, there are several recurring themes:

- Need—to "do and do and do" for the children to make up for their disability. Dr. Haim Ginott, in *Between Parent and Child*, wrote:

  For me a child's laughter and his tears have equal importance. I would not want to take away from him disappointment, sorrow, grief. Emotions enoble character. The deeper we feel, the more human we become . . . They can grow from the experience as long as you don't pollute it for them.

  Dr. Ginnott did not say that suffering builds character. But he did remind parents that feelings are part of our humanness. Mothers cannot make everything all right when it is not. Mothers CAN nurture potential, set necessary limits, establish realistic and challenging expectations, and work toward developing their children's sense of self-worth.

- Anger—at physicians who did not listen; nurses who were judgmental; and medical personnel in general, who were insensitive—Dr. Mary Robinson, Director of Child Life at the Children's Hospital National Medical Center in Washington D.C. tells young physicians: "While you will become experts on children, I hope you will always remember that parents are the experts on their own child."

  Mothers need to develop a "therapeutic alliance" with the professionals who care for their children. Sometimes physicians do not listen, nurses are quick to judge, and careless staff fail to respond in a helpful manner. A confident, knowledgeable mother will be able to express her discomfort and work toward improving relationships.

  Mothers coping with sick children need to deal with the issues at hand so they can move on to the next need. This is not advice to "keep a stiff upper lip." It is more a reminder of the classic prayer that asks for serenity to accept what can't be changed, courage to tackle what can, and wisdom to distinguish between the two.

Parent support groups in the hospital, where staff and parents come together to discuss the children's health and illness, hospital policy and rules, and families' needs, have helped reduce some of the tensions that develop out of such communication problems.

It is crucial that mothers become informed consumers. Know all you should about your child's condition. Keep records so you can give a good history, and stand your ground when you feel you must and your child's best interest is on the line.

- Helplessness and frustration—The red tape of admissions and insurance; the time wasted waiting at pharmacies and in doctors' offices; the children's bad dispositions—is it their temperament or their illness?, etc., etc.

Sometimes the hospital social services department can step in and straighten out complicated procedures and problems. If you have not been visited by a hospital social worker, you would be wise to make an appointment to see what assistance that department can offer, even if your children were discharged months ago. Also, speak to the doctors if they are part of the problem; even if they aren't, tell them of your difficulties and ask for their advice.

If it turns out that your frustrations are going to have to be part of your life, look for ways to offset them. Mothers suggest reading books and attending parenting workshops in the community or in the hospital; you may find that where your children's behavior is concerned or childrearing problems are at issue, your children are just behaving like their peers. If it's time management that is a problem, mothers have found that there are others who can wait for prescriptions at pharmacies, and help with such things as car pooling and meeting commitments.

You, as a mother, must first identify WHICH of the frustrations are most irritating before you can take the necessary steps to eliminate them. Then you have to define WHAT sort of help would ease those feelings of helplessness.

- Loss of identity—"I don't feel like a woman." "I'm too tired to be a good mother." "Who wants a wife that looks like this?" "All I do is play nurse—give medicines, change appliances, and drive to the doctor." Women build for themselves ideal images of good wives, good mothers, long-suffering mothers. But when it becomes necessary suddenly to be all those things, and the experience turns out to be one of anger and resentment, they may long for another identity—or at least wonder how they are going to juggle all their roles. From the outside it may look as if they ought to be sanctified before the week is out. On the inside they may be dying.

There is no easy answer, only the reminder that these are the sentiments of many, many mothers, including those whose children have had nothing more than one ear infection, one cold, and the chicken pox.

This unsettling loss of identity, experienced by so many new mothers and mothers of toddlers, is common enough to have generated postpartum neighborhood support groups, where new mothers and their babies come together to share common interests and concerns. You don't have to have a sick child to have mother-worries.

■ Fear of the future—"Will this mean that Tom can't be on the police force?" "How will Melissa ever be attractive to boys?" "School?" "Camp?" The questions come quickly and the need for answers seems urgent. What other group of mothers thinks to ask the pediatrician about the future sex life of their two-day-old infants? Did you ask if your four-year-old would be able to go skiing or be a cheerleader?

The larger concern that leads to such questions is, of course, quality of life. What sort of quality will your children's growing up have? No one can give you the answers, at least not certain answers; but you have every right to ask the questions and to mull over in your mind what sort of compromises you and other members of your family will have to make. This is a necessary and useful part of looking at your family traditions and values, and realigning them into harmony with this unwelcomed and unexpected event—your children's birth defect or illness. But be warned that if you are asking such questions amid the beeps and bleeps of high technology in a pediatric intensive care unit, the staff may answer curtly or ignore what they consider to be an outlandish inquiry. Remember that their immediate priority is to keep your children alive, not to raise them.

■ Isolation from friends and neighbors—Whether it's the birth of an infant with an abnormality or a dreadfully ill teenager, it can be shocking to friends and neighbors. They do not know how or what to say. They may first imagine how they would feel, and find themselves with a loss for words. Many find it easier to stay away. Others will rush to your side and utter such "dumb" and offensive sentiments that you will push them away.

Of course they do not mean to add to your pain, but sometimes they can seem insensitive. More than one mother can recall writing sad letters to friends, telling of their children's serious illness and the possibility that they might die. The friends might send back messages of consolation, with such supportive statements as "Yes, death might be a blessed relief . . ." By the time their notes arrived, the gravely ill child was putting together a model in the playroom. The peril had passed, but the friendship may have been permanently damaged.

Some mothers find relief in talking about their children's illnesses and their experiences with them, and talking, and talking, and talking . . . It may be a way to wind down and defuse, but it also can be a way to turn away friends, and eventually to eliminate telephone calls of concern. None will be as interested in the vivid details as you are. A few will indulge you in the beginning, because they understand your need to "talk it out." Even the most devoted, however, will not be marathon listeners forever.

■ Difficulty in adjusting to their children's wellness after surgery—As unusual as this sounds, as perverse as it may seem to mothers who are struggling with children who are anticipating surgery, the fact is that being the mother of a sick child becomes a way of life and a way of thinking. The schedule of activities is busy, usually hectic. The time for neighborhood, community, and even other family events is reduced. The children who are ill are likely to be calm and compliant, even lethargic. Even perfectly well children who are incontinent of urine realize their dependency on their mothers for dry pads and support in social situations.

After surgery things are likely to be quite different. Children are thrilled at their new freedom. Many feel they ought to make up for lost time, even when they're only seven. Mothers find it difficult to "let go" after being so attentive for such a long time. "And," as one admitted, "I have to tell you there were times I really missed my excuse. Sandy's requirements had excused me from taking my turn at the school cafeteria, from fixing dinners after a tough day at the hospital, getting the wash done, and keeping up with chores. Of course, I was thrilled that Sandy's surgery had been such a success. But, I wouldn't be honest if I didn't admit that sometimes it was hard for me."

Mothers, if they are average mothers, suffer with their children—whether it's poison ivy, a broken leg, or a terrible disease or deformity. The degree of misery is affected by the children's condition, the mothers' understanding and attitudes about it, and existing support systems. Just staying as flexible as possible is important, because children's demands—in sickness and in good health—shift and change continuously.

No one will tell you that caring for children with ostomies is going to be easy. But some will tell you that it is less difficult than caring for children with diabetes, epilepsy, or cardiac problems; in fact, many mothers of such other children will view your problems as minor compared to theirs. What everyone may tell you, whether or not you want to hear it, is that you must not permit the situation to be blown out of proportion and to become worse than it really is. If you are hearing such advice repeatedly from your husband, your parents, or members of the medical staff, pause and take stock. Your children can only judge themselves by your reflections. Are you reflecting reasonable confidence, optimism, and determination?

Fathers

Fathers often are thought to be most concerned about their children's ability to play sports, get a manly job, and "grow up to be a chip off the old block"—an unfair caricature of men, who grieve as deeply as women when their babies are malformed or their sons and daughters become ill and require major body alterations. For most fathers, the concerns are no less; they are just different:

■ Disappointment and anger—Often, they say, their anger is not so much at what has occurred but at what the events symbolize. Like, ". . . I always thought I was supposed to take care of her, but now look what's happened." It's as if some fathers feel they should have been able to prevent the problem or, at the least, make it go away. Somehow they feel they have failed to meet their obligations of husbandhood and fatherhood.

Fathers who tend to think analytically simply KNOW that this sort of tragedy should not happen, and become angry when no one can explain it so they can understand. One exasperated parent stood defiantly listening to an ET describe ulcerative colitis, the numerous theories about it that have come to naught, and the continued quest for the cause of the disease that had sapped his son's strength, energy, and good humor. "Well," he sputtered, "this is a hell of a way to run a railroad. I can tell you that my company wouldn't last five minutes if we couldn't find the cause of our problems. I'm in construction and if our buildings started crumbling, I can assure you that we would devote the time and energy to get to the source of the defect and correct it." You can hear the frustration and anger that this man feels, to think that brilliant minds in medicine and science, for all these years, have been unable to find the cause of inflammatory bowel disease.

- Occupational conflicts—Shift work, travel, and frequent transfers are job requirements that interfere with caring for sick children. Some fathers want very much to participate, but feel they cannot jeopardize their family's financial security by requesting a job with no travel, or asking not to be moved to another city. One father said, "There I was trying to protect our income, that was going to be a drop in the bucket of medical bills, and the boss says, 'You're just going to have to decide what is important.' I used to drive 190 miles a day and every one of 'em was spent trying to decide, until I realized that it was like giving a guy a choice between the guillotine and the electric chair."

  Other fathers hearing this story nodded sympathy, but two men said they were locked into their company because of the benefit package; they just had to bargain, and bank on compassionate supervisors. One father told of considering a job change that would mean more money immediately and in the future; but, under the new company's health and benefit package, his daughter would be excluded. No amount of salary would be sufficient for the medical bills she might well incur in the years ahead. Fathers in the military have had to request assignments to locations with adequate treatment facilities, and to refuse assignments to areas where their career might have advanced at the expense of their children's health or treatment needs.

- What did I do wrong? An affair, a fight, premarital sex? Particularly when they have a son whose genitalia is deformed, men have sometimes felt like it was a punishment for their misdeeds. One distraught father was convinced it was retribution for the "wild" life he had led as a teenager in rural Iowa. The problem was that he had to suffer in silence, because when his wife had met him she had had the impression that he had always been a well-behaved, upstanding, church-going boy. Until he squared his past with his wife, no amount of counseling could make him feel better or convince him that his guilt was misplaced. When he finally confessed, his wife laughed with relief that his escapades had not been more serious. Together they were able to forge a stronger personal relationship, as well as a partnership in the care of their son.

- Bills to pay—There are many combinations of stark terror and resentment over medical indebtedness. Men are embarrassed or bitter that the hospital bills are so much more than they earn or than their insurance companies will pay. They may resent the loss of income when a wife has to give up work to care for their child. Men have been saving for retirement, frills, or college tuition for their children and see their accounts wiped clean. Imagine looking in the mirror every morning and thinking that, no matter how hard you work, how many hours you work, you will never be able to get out of debt!

Money can be a terribly important factor, and the financial situation should be faced as effectively as possible. Fathers are encouraged to take time off from their job, as soon as they can after their children's problem has been discovered, to explore every possible means of financial assistance. A meeting with the company personnel department, an appointment with the social service department in the hospital, a call to state and local agencies, a meeting with the physicians and the hospital billing department—this sort of exploration will take time but it may well make all the difference, between getting medical care without cutting into the basic family budget, and embarking on a treatment plan that will devastate the bank account.

■ Unwillingness to accept responsibility—As some young (and not so young) fathers have confessed (after listening to surgeons outlining their children's condition, proposed surgery, prognosis): "I just couldn't handle it. Here I was in the prime of life. A job to get done, a future, good friends that were ready to have fun, and a good-looking wife. All of a sudden I have to stay up half the night with a sick kid, do the grocery shopping and run errands after work, come home to a wife who's either at the hospital or at home too tired from her day at the hospital to pay attention to me. And who can go out with friends when you can't even get a babysitter? I just told my wife it was too much."

It's easy to denounce such fathers; but it is also easy to empathize with their realistic appraisal of a very tough situation. One father said in bewilderment: "For my wife, our child's sickness just meant a big job made bigger. For me it added another full-time job to the one I was already working."

■ Fear—More attention is being given to father's first hours and days with their infants, and the effects on later parenting. There is increasing research evidence suggesting that they establish a closer bond if they have spent more time holding and caring for their infants. But a 2½ pound premature infant in an isolette is a terrifying sight to most people; and it may be particularly frightening to a father who only recently agreed to change diapers, after being pressured by other males in the Lamaze classes.

Standing over children who have tubes running in and out of every cavity, and who look as white as their sheets, many fathers have feared their children would die as they stood there; feared they would cause their death by touching something they shouldn't, as they tried to touch their children; feared they might throw up at the sight of the stoma, or blood, or whatever made them queasy.

But there is help. Sensitive nurses and physicians will welcome fathers to neonatal units, and stay with them until they have gained confidence and comfort in the mechanistic and forbidding environment.

In part because they are off at work when the doctors' offices, clinics, and ancillary services are open, men's feelings often go unnoticed and unattended. If this entire book did nothing more than make one father more comfortable with his child, or one reader more aware of the special hurts and needs of fathers of sick children, it would have been worthwhile.

Couples

Couples who stand before a justice of the peace or a church altar (or who choose not to) do so with many intentions and promises. Only a rare couple, who makes the headlines or the 6 o'clock news, can say that the partners entered a relationship with the knowledge that there would be sadness, tragedy, hurt, physical and mental anguish, and disagreement. Author K. C. Cole criticizes parenting books that tell people that "IF they do this, that or the other, THEN they are assured a predictable outcome."

In marriage partnerships, with or without children, this is a foolish expectation that certainly must account, in part, for the rampant divorce rate. Where there are children to care for, their presence guarantees a certain degree of disharmony and stress—no matter how lovable or healthy they are.

A teacher in a San Diego High School was most creative in demonstrating the demands a child makes on a marriage. Her students paired off as couples. Each pair was given a raw egg, which simulated a fragile child. The two were responsible for this raw egg for a week. Like a child, it could not be left alone. At the end of the exercise a crack in the egg signified illness or injury. A broken egg symbolized death.

Some fashioned string carriers around their neck or special holders for a book bag or bike. One can only imagine what a couple did to safeguard their egg when one was at football practice and the other was practicing her cheers.

The lesson was effective. The teenagers became aware of the kinds of plans necessary to safeguard one small egg. It wasn't hard for them to envision the sorts of sacrifices and attention required for a dependent human being.

Couples bring to their union many expectations that they have discussed during their courtship, as well as many they harbor subconsciously, or just assume their partner understands. Some of these expectations come from their cultural heritage, their education, their own parents' behavior, books, movies, fantasy, and, of course, prevailing sex-role stereotypes.

Sometimes when young couples who have not been together long have an infant with a deformity, their problems are amplified because they haven't yet clarified their roles and expectations in the partnership. Who does the supper dishes? Who changes the toilet paper roll, walks the dog, buys the booze, empties the garbage, pays the bills, talks to the landlord, sends parents birthday cards? Before they have had a chance to sort out and agree on these responsibilities, they are coping with the requirements of a child who demands many decisions and hours of care.

Other couples may hope that a baby will strengthen a frail marriage. The baby arrives with multiple problems that only complicate the troubles—and the situation gets worse.

As couples who have had one can tell you, there is never a right time to have a catastrophe. It is no less stressful when men and women have been married for a number of years and a growing, lively child becomes desperately ill, wrecking childhood fantasies and family plans. There are some poignant stories that merit sharing, of couples who have grappled with their children's disabilities.

Mr. and Mrs. D. had been married for seven years. Mr. D was nearly a decade older than his wife. They had wanted to start their family early, and Mrs. D. had been terribly upset when she didn't conceive in the first two years. Then she became pregnant. But two miscarriages followed. Finally, a beautiful baby girl was born; and two long, frustrating years later a baby boy was born, with bladder exstrophy. Within a year the couple's marriage had disintegrated into a stilted, polite relationship "for the children's sake." Mr. D. complained that all his wife did was take care of their son. Mrs. D. said that all her husband did was take their beautiful little girl on fun outings.

As they finally sifted through their problems and identified their feelings and accusations, these were some of the emotions they were able to express:

Hers: *Necessity to provide ALL her son's care, to demonstrate her superior ability in child care since she had not demonstrated such success in conceiving or carrying children.*

Necessity to provide ALL her son's care because the sight of his malformed genitalia would be too painful for her husband.

Jealousy that her husband preferred to take their daughter on outings, and that the two of them were developing such a close relationship.

Suspicion that her husband's advanced age was the cause of their son's problem. (Mr. D. was 38 when Paul was born. Presumably, his wife had not read about Bing Crosby's second family, Senator Strom Thurmond of South Carolina, and Charlie Chaplin.)

Terror at the thought of ever getting pregnant again.

His: *Rejection as a father because he was never allowed to participate in his son's care.*

Rejection as a husband because his wife had no time for him.

Pity for their daughter and determination to make certain that she would not feel neglected like he did.

Concern that his wife thought him unmanly because she blamed "weak sperm" for her miscarriages and Paul's deformity.

Imagine trying to function as individuals or parents with such misconceptions and faulty communications. Fortunately, they got help. Shortly after they began participating in a parents' group they were able to begin working on rebuilding their relationship.

Unforgettable was the couple that waited outside the operating room during the six hours their daughter was inside. The mother was seated bolt upright for all 360 minutes. She smoked two packages of cigarettes, drank four Diet Pepsis, and ate a package of Fritos. She tried to read two magazines but couldn't concentrate. He delivered the first two soft drinks and chatted pleasantly with a couple of other parents who came and went. Finally, he decided he would make good use of his time and take a nap so he would be rested later. That's when the four-year-war started.

He believed he had just been sensible. She believed he had been callous. She had told him so when she had awakened him a half hour after he went to sleep, and she told him so at least once a week for the next 48 months. Their daughter felt guilty each time the subject came up, because she was now rid of her dreadful problem and well adjusted to her ostomy, while they were still suffering.

Men have been aghast and disgusted when their working wives have expressed their intent to continue working and have wanted to discuss such practical questions as how the two of them would share doctor's appointments and who would stay home with the children if they became ill. Wives have confessed bitter disappointment that their husbands went right back to work "as if nothing had happened."

Fortunately there have also been positive stories, of other parents who told of struggling together, and creating a marriage and a family that might never have had such dimension had it not been for their children's illnesses.

No one can give you a sure-fire prescription for safeguarding your relationship as a couple when one of your children has a serious health problem. But any good counsel will offer at least some of these messages:

■ Remember that different people react to stress in different ways.

■ Remember that different people show hurt, love and concern differently.

■ Listen to what your partner is saying and doing.

■ Learn to communicate with your mate. Seek counseling or an objective listener to help you talk to each other.

■ Don't use your child as an excuse or a weapon when the real problems have probably been smoldering for a long time.

■ Don't use your child as an excuse or a weapon—no matter what!

As the parent part of the family, whether you are male or female, single or married, in an original or blended constellation, you are first a person. Only when you are able to get your own person in order are you able to then function in your other roles as wife, husband, parent, etc. And you cannot "give up everything" for a sick child, because there will be nothing left to offer your child—except one tired, over-extended parent with an acute case of burn-out.

Siblings

Brothers and sisters have stories to tell, too—of confusion, loneliness, guilt, anger, etc. It can be helpful to remind yourself of the mental competencies and psychological tasks of your other children. Are they at the age where they may feel guilty thinking that something they did caused their sib's illness? Are they at the age that they are embarrassed to have a brother or sister who's "different," frightened that it will soon happen to them, or jealous of the attention another child is receiving? In an old but wonderful book, *What to Tell Your Child*, Helene Arnstein cautions, "Children tend to worry more about themselves if there's an aura of mystery surrounding their illness . . ." Yes, and siblings are liable to worry more, too, if doors are closed and folks whisper in hallways.

Imagine seeing a brother or sister walk out of the house, be gone for a period of time that you do not comprehend, and return with a suitcase full of toys, puzzles and new clothes. Imagine being told that you should forgive your brother when he took your toys, knocked down your castles, and colored in your books, and that you should never hit him back, because "he is sick."

Brothers and sisters may become hypochondriacs, and take to the bed or complain endlessly about minor symptoms or injuries; they may become stoic and hide any sign of illness for fear it will lead to something awful; they may start acting out their frustrations—from biting and hitting when they're young to drinking and using drugs when they're older.

Do not wait for them to send a signal that they too are suffering. Make early plans to help them cope—to compensate for attention they don't receive, time you can't spend with them, and responsibilities they may have to assume in a family in which a child is ill.

Teena Sorenson, a Parent Educator and psychiatric nurse from San Antonio, Texas, advises:

> The well-being of the siblings of handicapped children is influenced by factors such as their birth order in the family, their physical similarities to or differences from the handicapped child and the socioeconomic and cultural circumstances of the family. The severity of the handicap plays some part, though not a critical one. By far the most important factor is the adjustment of the parents to their situation, their feelings and their ability to support each other and to parent all of the children.

Grandparents

Grandparents may be a near or distant part of the family. Wherever they are, they are likely to play a major role, even when it's invisible.

People did not discuss bowels "when <u>they</u> were growing up." Sex wasn't a topic at the dinner table "when <u>they</u> were young." Now suddenly there's a child in the family whose condition is difficult to discuss without discussing one or both of these subjects.

Some grandparents grieve for their child's disappointment and secretly resent their grandchild for causing it. Some want to jump in and take over just as they would have when their child was little—to care and protect. John's mother told of her dilemma. When they would go visit Grandmother, she would reach right past Tommy, the little brother, to "poor John." Tommy no longer wanted to go visit Grandmother. And Grandmother indulged John with food, attention and gifts that made him "act rotten" for days afterwards.

Many women have a fantasy of what a grandmother should be, and how a grandfather, too, should act. They should be like they were in the first grade readers: kind, attentive, loving and available. In the 1980's they may not be available; they are liable to be hard at work, keeping a busy schedule at the Senior Citizen Center, or involved with their own circle of friends. They may well live across the country and have little understanding of their grandchild's illness or the help their children could use. They may never have heard of an ostomy, or, worse, they may have known someone in '25 or '43 who "had one of those things and suffered the tortures of the damned."

Sometimes invisible grandparents cause problems just by their absence, because of the resentment their apparent disinterest creates. On the other hand, it is a boon to families when grandparents can and will share chores and child care requirements.

Aunts, Uncles, and Cousins

Aunts, uncles and cousins play varying roles in today's family. Children with ostomies often spend their first night away from home, or make their first revelation about their ostomy at a cousin's house. Relatives' attitudes about and understanding of ostomies must be considered before judging their behavior toward your children. Include them where it is feasible and educate them however you can.

In Summary

The family is where people are formed. Virginia Satir writes: "I am convinced there are no genes to carry the feeling of worth. It is learned and the family is where it is learned." Mrs. Satir has identified the characteristics she consistently finds in families where loving, creative, and productive human beings are nurtured:

■ Self-worth is high;

■ Communication is direct, clear, specific and honest;

■ Rules are flexible, humane, appropriate and subject to change; and

■ The linking to society is open and hopeful.

Many men and women bumble through parenthood doing the best they can, and do a fine job. Young people, without guidebooks to refer to, grow up in spite of their parents as well as because of them. When children are born with disabilities, sustain a terrible injury, or acquire a serious illness, parents usually are forced to assess their values and consciously design strategies for child rearing. This greater emphasis on planning may bring satisfaction and effectiveness not possible with the "by guess or by gosh" approach. When asked to account for his obvious success, a handsome quadriplegic said, "Oh, it was my parents. They treated me just like I was normal." After a thoughtful pause he added, "And now that I'm older I realize just how hard that must have been for them."

When all subjects have been covered, anatomy lessons learned, and ostomy management techniques honed, parents return again to the persistent question, "Can we do anything to help our children accept the problems they must live with?" Dr. Lee Salk concludes,*

> Yes. You can recognize, and help them recognize, that problems are relative . . . It is easier for your children to live with problems if they accept them as a normal part of normal life. In fact, problem-solving adds zest to life. Of course, it helps your children to know that you want to help them with their problems. You should let your children know that you care about them, that you will be there to help them when they need you. Make them understand that their feelings concern you, that you enjoy them as they are, together with their problems. In short, that you love them as they are. Believe me, when your children see you expressing love like this, they will learn from you to love. After all, didn't you learn to live with some of your problems? And, in spite of them, don't you give and receive love? To look at it another way, who wants to know the perfect human being? Or, worse yet, to be the perfect human being? It would be a terrible responsibility, and it would be impossible to find anyone who would love you.

*What Every Child Would Like His Parents to Know, New York, David McKay (1972).

About Neighbors, Teachers and Classmates

As young children venture from home, their outside social experiences begin first in the front yard, then expand through the neighborhood, and finally extend to the classroom. Neighbors, teachers and classmates are among the first people to whom most children must explain their ostomies. There will be many different reactions—curiosity, pity, disgust, rejection and nonchalant acceptance.

The surer children are that they are loveable, the less security they will need from their environment. If a strong sense of personal worth has been nurtured at home, they will be more secure in a group. Children with ostomies will be teased just because children will be teased. (In fact, the absence of teasing, or of not being noticed at all, can be as upsetting as taunting or name calling.) But a strong self-image will be of great help when the criticism comes.

Neighbors

Parents ask early what they should do about the neighbors—How to tell them. What to tell them. Although there is no one "best" solution, here is advice offered by mothers over the years:

- We didn't tell any of our neighbors because we didn't want them to treat our child differently. Neither did we keep it a secret. When there was a reason to confide, like a sleepover or several families going away together, then we explained. Boy, were people impressed!

- We told the parents of our child's best friends so they would understand if we seemed a little "hyper" about the rules. We asked them to let us know if they ever detected an odor or our child made a mess in the bathroom.

- Everybody in the neighborhood knows. After all, our child has had numerous hospitalizations and the neighbors have been part of the family. They've cooked, cleaned, babysat and broken up fights!

- Most of the neighbors have just come to know about it over the years. We've had to speak to a few who were being overprotective and hollering at their children not to tease or play rough with ours. That was hard because we knew they were only trying to be kind.

■ We had never said much to our neighbors, one way or the other. Our son was testing an appliance for a company. The pouch was bright blue and he loved it. He went to at least five of the mothers in the neighborhood and said, "Look at the new bag I got today!" My phone didn't stop ringing for three days.

Most parents concur that secrecy creates more curiosity and rumors than anything else, but that telling everyone right away isn't always the answer either. "In time you just know when it's appropriate to mention it."

Mothers agree that there is one thing, above all others, that makes caring for children with ostomies difficult. When the children are dressed, and they have no other disabilities, it's hard to imagine that they've ever been sick a day. One mother said, "You try not to ever mention it around new neighbors or friends who don't know; but, then, it's really hard to avoid telling people about the awful things you've been through and what a hero your child is. It's almost like it would be easier if everybody could SEE, and then they'd UNDERSTAND why things are like they are and we're the way we are."

Mothers who have participated in activities of the United Ostomy Association have agreed that this is where they've found the most support. Said an enthusiastic mother, "It's a wonderful group that knows what you're talking about and can relate to your experiences, even if they're not parents of children with ostomies but ostomates themselves."

Teachers

Oh, the stories mothers tell about teachers! Poor teachers. They deserve special consideration in this text because, when it comes to dealing with children who have ostomies, many wear several hats. As classroom leaders they must think of the whole class, the 28 or so other pupils. Many times children who are hospital vets are accustomed to more individualized and frequent attention. They find sharing a teacher and working according to class rules difficult. Also those who are away from attentive mothers for the first time may be disruptive.

Most teachers in elementary schools are female. Many are mothers, too. It is hard for some of them not to show pity and preferential treatment for a "special child" in their classroom, even when that child looks just like all the others. Some teachers' protective nature has gotten the best of them. They've made up their own rules that set children apart, and they've gathered the class together to tell them about their "special" classmate. (You will remember that ostomate children themselves have said that they are the ones who should do the explaining.)

Teachers, too, often are aware of their role as part of the school administration and, in that role, become safety conscious. They fear that bending rules or procedures for one may lead to school anarchy. It may be amusing to read about; it's hardly humorous when parents report that children's crutches have been moved out of reach; that children have been advised not to take gym; and that teachers have restricted bathroom privileges.

Mrs. A. summed it up to a parents group: "Sometimes even the mildest parents have to be fighters [for their children]." Before parents wage war or begin their campaign, however, it may be helpful for them to pause to consider the teachers' side—that is, which of their multiple roles is influencing the particular actions and decisions.

Regular parent-teacher conferences can be very helpful.

In all but unusual circumstances, parents of children with ostomies should not ask teachers to function as their children's nurse, too.

Classmates

Nearly all parents yearn to shield and spare their children. But there is virtually nothing effective that parents can do outside the home. On the other hand, they can be enormously effective inside the home, by nurturing their children's self-esteem. Parents can demonstrate to their children by their early acceptance that having an ostomy is not a shameful thing. They can help their children formulate explanations to playmates and friends, encourage association with role models when the age is appropriate, set limits and nurture self-reliance.

Non-conforming youngsters who act up in school are not likely to enjoy success. According to Audrey McCollum in *Coping With Prolonged Health Impairment In Your Child*, "No child whose behavior frequently arouses anger and resentment in those around him—reactions he readily senses—can develop a secure sense of personal worth."

Some ideas mothers have offered:

■ We made simple line drawings for our child that illustrated his conditions so other kids could understand.

- We sat our child down when he was three and said, "Now look, you are going to explain your ostomy to your playmates and friends so they know why you go to the toilet differently."

- For a health class assignment we encouraged our son to write an essay about ostomy. His classmates were fascinated. He had no trouble explaining after that.

- We told our 13-year-old daughter that she should get used to handling her ostomy now—in gym, at sleep-overs, etc.—if she ever intended to go away to college.

It is written so often that children are cruel. Is it not their honesty that is often so cruel? Getting along with classmates is essential to social growth and progress toward maturity. Classmates become increasingly important to children's emerging body image and self-esteem. It is important that they measure up—physically, socially and academically—or be able to compensate where they are not able.

Among other responses, classmates may actually be envious. Many have reacted as one in particular did: "Wow, you mean you can just pull that plug anytime, anywhere? You don't even have to get up in the night or look for a toilet? What luck!"

As Erik Erikson has said, "School is a culture all of its own." You, as parents, can only prepare them to take their place among their classmates, and help cultivate the interpersonal skills necessary to be successful there.

Notes

Conditions That Lead to Ostomies

Most parents ask first, "Is the baby all right? Are all ten fingers and toes there?" Thinking about the number of systems in the human body and their complexity makes one quickly realize that it is amazing that most of them do always work "on delivery," and continue in good working order for sixty to eighty years with very little maintenance or attention. The two systems involved when ostomies are discussed are the gastrointestinal (digestive) and genitourinary tracts. Parts of them may be put to rest temporarily, or discarded if they cannot be repaired; but they both are vitally important to the processes of nourishment, growth, and elimination of waste products.

The Digestive System

Consider first the digestive system. (Figure 37) The process of digestion begins in the mouth where teeth chew the food, and enzymes in the saliva do the initial processing. Chewing is important because the digestive juices can act more efficiently on smaller particles. (The baby-food-makers have helped out where teeth have not come in.) Swallowing passes the mashed material into the esophagus, where it is propelled to the stomach by peristalsis, a rhythmical squeezing motion. Further digestion occurs in the stomach by means of a mechanical churning action and the chemical action of enzymes and acids that act on the food received.

The food passes out of the stomach, now in a more liquid form and full of enzymes, and into the small intestine. Two important processes occur here. Juices from the pancreas and liver further the digestive process by breaking down foods into simple sugars, amino acids, and fatty acids, utilizing bacteria specifically adapted to the task.* The portion of digested products the body can use passes through the walls of the small intestine to nurture the body. (Remember that the small intestine would be a very long pipe if it were not coiled as it is in the abdomen.) The residue is conveyed into the large intestine.

*There are many kinds of bacteria in the intestinal tract. (Nature is amazing because the type and amount are carefully balanced. Too few, too many, or "foreign invaders" may cause illness.)

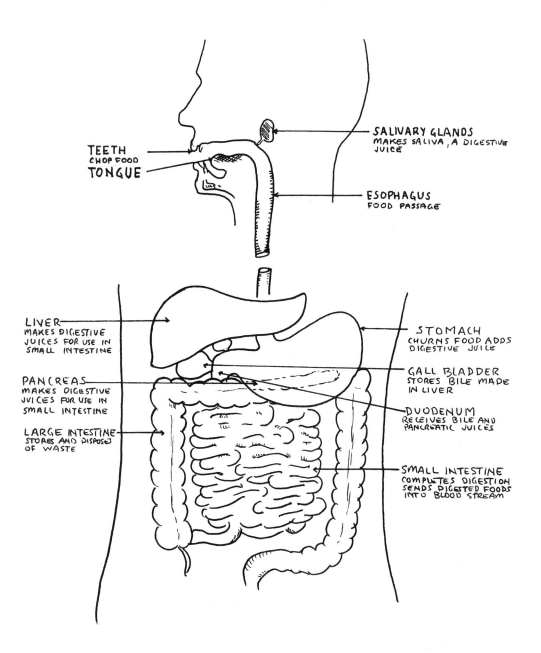

FIGURE 31   **THE DIGESTIVE SYSTEM**

The functions of the large intestine are to absorb water and minerals (for use by the body); and to transport the food residue that are no longer useful to the rectum.

In infancy evacuation is produced by a reflex that usually is triggered shortly after feeding. Later, control of the reflex is the key to passage of stool at a convenient time and a proper place. Most parents were taught when they were children that a formed stool once or twice daily is normal and necessary.

Dr. Denis Burkitt of England has done vast research in Africa and other developing countries in recent years and has demonstrated that children and adults who consume a diet high in natural fibre have more stools that are of softer consistency and greater volume. He believes that such a diet protects people from diseases of the colon that are common among Americans and in other Western cultures. Not everyone agrees with Dr. Burkitt.

In Western societies toilet training is an important part of growing up, and the earlier it can be accomplished the happier most parents (and children) will be. When children do not achieve bowel control by the age of three or three-and-one-half, a number of predictable events occur: trips to doctors in search of anatomical problems, family fights, and outbursts of frustration and rage when daily soiling and foul-smelling pants require extra laundry chores, baths, and explanations to curious relatives and friends.

At the end of the digestive tract, which also is called the alimentary canal, are the rectum and finally the anus that opens to the outside of the body. The anal sphincter is the amazing purse-string mechanism that can let gases out while keeping solid matter in, and that can be kept tightly shut until it is released, at will, by the person in control. Damage to or absence of the sphincter means that bowel movements will be difficult or impossible to control.

The Genitourinary System

The genitourinary system, like the gastrointestinal tract, has several parts, each performing specific tasks. (Figure 38) Picture the kidneys as a filtration plant. They extract waste from blood delivered to them via the renal artery, and return cleansed blood to circulation. The waste products become urine. Adults produce a quart or so of urine a day from the filtering of some 50 gallons of blood plasma. An infant's bladder holds approximately 1½ to 3 ounces of urine; most adults are able to store somewhere between 8-12 ounces before voiding.

Kidneys are essential to life. Most people are born with two. Occasionally a person will have just one. Some people will have multiple or horseshoe kidneys. Even a single damaged kidney can sustain a normal life in some circumstances.

The urine that is formed in the kidneys is transported by peristalsis down pipes, called ureters, for storage in the bladder. When the bladder has reached its capacity, the urge to void is signalled. When the bladder neck opens, the urine passes through the uretha to the outside. A complicated network of communications between brain, nerves, and muscles determines how well the bladder holds urine without overflowing, holding too much, or simply emptying unexpectedly.

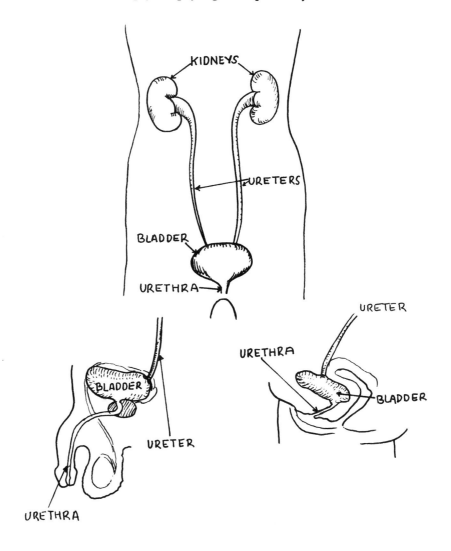

FIGURE 38   THE GENITOURINARY SYSTEM

The urinary tract, in normal condition, is always sterile. Infection is one signal that something is not working correctly.

The parts of the urinary system that transport and store urine may be bypassed or removed if they are diseased or deformed, and life will not be endangered as long as a satisfactory substitute is made; but a certain amount of kidney tissue is essential for a person to grow and be well. Without it the only solutions are the regular use of an artificial kidney (dialysis) or a kidney transplant.

In the male, the reproductive system is part of the urinary system. (That explains the prefix "genito" you have seen several times.) Sperm are made in the testes that reside in the scrotum and come up tubes called the "vas deferens" and merge with semen and prostatic fluid to be transported through the urethra out the tip of the penis during ejaculation. In females the reproductive system and urinary tract are separate. (Figure 39).

With just this basic information it will be easier for you to understand the birth defects that occur in these systems and the diseases that lead to ostomies.

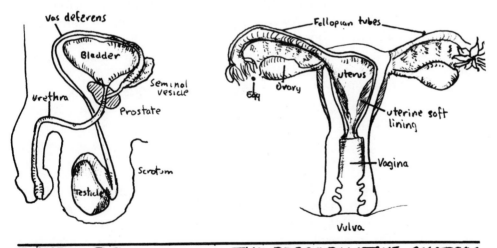

FIGURE 39   THE REPRODUCTIVE SYSTEM

Problems in the Gastrointestinal Tract

Neonatal necrotizing enterocolitis. Breaking that difficult series of words into understandable living-room conversation only takes a minute. *Neonatal* means newborn. *Necrosis* refers to the death of tissues or organs and *necrotizing* to dying. *Colitis* means an inflammation of the colon. Putting all this back together in simple language you may say, "A portion of the bowel is dead." This means that nothing can pass through the intestine at this point. Even more serious, though, is the fact that dead tissue is not tolerated by the body.

Neonatal necrotizing enterocolitis, sometimes called NEC or NNE around hospital wards and clinics, occurs in 3-8% of premature infants. It is most common in newborns who weigh less than three pounds.

The diagnosis may be made as early as the first day of life, or not for a week or two. Many of these babies can be saved by removing the gangrenous (another way of saying dead) piece of bowel and performing an ileostomy. As soon as the baby gets big and healthy enough to withstand another operation, the ileostomy can be closed and the intestines will function normally.

When people see Christopher today it is hard to imagine that he ever was a three-pound wonder. He was so little that most appliances looked like he was meant to be put in them, rather than they on him. Special pouches are made for tiny "premies."

Imperforate Anus. Recall that the anus is the opening where the large intestine connects with the outside of the body. *Perforate* means to make a hole in. *Imperforate*, then, means that there is no hole in something. Imperforate anus describes the absence of an exit for the bowel. There are several variations of the deformity and the severity depends upon where the colon stops inside the body.

Many children with imperforate anus live with a colostomy for approximately the first year of life, by which time the problem can be corrected surgically. Some have their colostomy longer, and a few are never able to achieve satisfactory bowel control, and keep their colostomy permanently.

Bev, a beautiful young lady, was one of the latter. She wanted her troublesome rectum removed before she married. She found that several surgeons didn't want to do that because it would eliminate any future possibility that the ostomy could be reversed. Bev remembered the attempts to repair her anal sphincter that had not been successful and assured them that she preferred the colostomy. The surgery was done in plenty of time for her to feel good as new before her wedding day.

It is not uncommon for babies with imperforate anus to have some urologic problems too. For this reason their physical examinations usually include tests and X-rays to identify any urinary abnormalities.

Cloacal exstrophy. The cloaca is the body cavity where the urinary, gastrointestinal, and generative organs come together. Exstrophy of the cloaca is the complicated deformity that results when the abdominal wall does not come together and intestinal and urinary organs are exposed on the outside of the body. Unfortunately, it is not just a matter of putting them back inside and closing the abdomen. Many infants will require both an ileostomy and a urostomy.

Jimmy was a little boy who needed to have an ileostomy and a ureterostomy (Figure 17, p. 28) from each kidney, to serve until he was older and his urologist would be able to make a urine system that required only one stoma. It was necessary to design a special belt to hold both the ileostomy and urostomy appliances in place.

The internal and external sex organs are affected too. Boys will have some degree of deformity of their penis and will require surgery to improve its appearance and the way it functions. Girls, too, will have abnormalities of their genitalia (the external sex organs). Pediatric urologists and plastic surgeons have done masterful jobs of repairing the problems. When the pubic hair grows in, this helps to improve the appearance even more.

When there are internal abnormalities, hormone treatment may be required at the onset of puberty. Such conditions are discussed with parents early, so they don't come as a surprise when the children reach their teens.

Hirschsprung's Disease. This is a defect that occurs most often in the descending colon, and it is not visible when the baby is born. Nerves, called the ganglion nerves, are missing, and stool doesn't pass through the abnormal section. Because it is not a visible abnormality, flu-like symptoms or prolonged or repeated bouts of constipation may lead to the diagnosis. A biopsy, in which a tiny snip of tissue from the bowel wall is taken using a colonoscope, will confirm the diagnosis.

Symptoms may not arise immediately after birth. Sometimes babies have colic-type problems for a long while before anyone looks for something more severe. An ileostomy or colostomy may be required to permit the passage of stool above the diseased portion of the intestine, or to protect the place where the damaged part is removed and the two normal ends of the bowel are rejoined.

Inflammatory bowel disease. This term (or sometimes IBD) is used when people are talking about granulomatous and ulcerative colitis, two distinctly different diseases that have many of the same symptoms. Granulomatous colitis is, along with ileitis and regional enteritis, referred to as Crohn's Disease.* It may be found anywhere along the alimentary canal.

---

*After Dr. Burrill Crohn who first described a granulomatous condition in 1932. Before that, the symptoms now called regional enteritis or Crohn's colitis were thought to represent tuberculosis or some other disease.

Ulcerative colitis (or CUC, for chronic ulcerative colitis) is confined usually to the large intestine; occasionally the end of the small intestine is involved. When it cannot be controlled with medicines, it can be cured by removing the large intestine and the rectum and performing an ileostomy. There is a high incidence of cancer among patients who have had active ulcerative colitis for more than ten years. This is not the case with Crohn's disease.

Inflammatory bowel disease occurs most commonly between the ages of 15 and 35, but others of all ages may suffer from it too. The common symptoms of both ulcerative and granulomatous colitis are frequent bloody stools, abdominal cramps, diarrhea, weight loss, and low grade fever. Fistulae, which are abnormal openings between two hollow organs or a hollow organ and the skin, may happen in Crohn's disease but are rare in ulcerative colitis.

Inflammatory bowel disease may be accompanied by complications outside the intestinal tract. It is not uncommon for patients to have arthritis, skin disorders, ulcers in the mouth like canker sores, and irritation in the eyes. No one understands fully the connection between these symptoms and the primary disease. Thankfully, for some they do not occur and for others they are not severe when they do.

One of the problems which can tip the scales in favor of surgery, is growth failure. For many youngsters of course, being abnormally small is a source of embarrassment in itself. And even though they weren't certain that an ileostomy was going to be a good thing, Tom and Marilyn said they both looked forward to the promise that they would begin to grow once they got rid of their diseased organs. Both heartily agreed, after their surgery, that it was great to be feeling good enough to be with their gang again; but they were most thrilled over catching up in size.

In 1981 the cause of these diseases is still unknown. Some families have had more than one member affected.

Because of the nature of the symptoms, it is only natural that they are confused with a whole host of problems, some more mental than physical. Even doctors can be misled, and may inquire whether the children are "hyper," or whether there is stress at school or at home. You've heard the old adage, "Don't get your bowels in an uproar"—suggesting that, if we calm down, our gut will too. One mother described her meeting with a new doctor: "I was as pleasant as I could be and did everything I could think of not to look like a colitic mother." Who knows what "colitic mothers" look or act like? But they have been described in textbooks as domineering and overbearing, tense and nagging.

It is hardly any wonder that patients with acute inflammatory bowel disease, and mothers who agonize with them, are likely to become tense, fatigued, nervous, unable to make friends easily. No wonder all the other terms and labels have been put on them, with all of the pain of the abdominal symptoms, the weight loss, the explosive diarrhea that may not wait for a toilet, and the massive doses of powerful medications.*

It generally is agreed now that stress may make the disease worse or cause it to flare up, but knowledgeable people no longer call it an "emotional disease." Guilt is the last thing parents need. It is counterproductive and tiring in itself. Don't fall into the trap and don't let anyone catch you up in it.

Problems of the Genitourinary Tract

The urinary system is formed about four months after a baby is conceived, and excretion begins before the baby is born. (The ears and the urinary tract are formed at about the same time and it is not uncommon for children with urologic disorders to have misshapen ears.) When there is an obstruction in the urinary tract that interferes with the flow of urine, the newborn may arrive with severe damage to the kidneys or other urinary organs.

Eagle-Barrett Syndrome (Prune Belly). This is an uncommon three-part birth defect which occurs in males. An absence of abdominal muscles causes the belly to look like a shriveled prune when the babies lie down. Thus the name "prune belly"—a very appropriate term, unless it's your baby. The other name, Eagle-Barrett Syndrome, which is used mostly by urologists in their medical journals, is after the men who first described the condition.

Besides the abdominal problem, the testicles are undescended and usually the urinary tract is in a condition known as *hydroureteronephrosis.*** This long word describes what has happened when urine has backed up and stretched the ureters and the kidneys out of shape. The bladder may be stretched too. That stretching (just like what happens to an elastic belt or girdle worn by a very fat person) damages the organs; so even when the urologist is able to fix the system, it may never be completely normal.

---

*Inge Tractenberg wrote an inspiring description of her family's ordeal with inflammatory bowel disease. Her book, *My Daughter, My Son,* describes, as only a mother could do, what it is like for children to suffer this condition and parents to suffer for and with them.

**This is another one of those words that must be divided into smaller parts. *Hydro-* refers to water; *uretero-* tells you the ureter, that pipe from the kidney to the bladder, is involved; *nephrosis* means a condition of the kidney.

The danger is that so much damage has been done before birth to the kidneys that the baby won't survive. It is easier to understand what has happened if you compare what hydroureteronephrosis looks like on an X-ray with what a normal X-ray of the urinary tract would look like. (Figure 40)

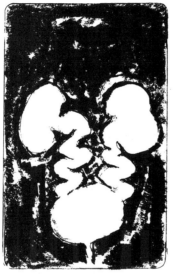

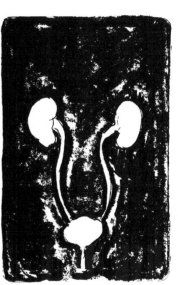

XRAY OF
HYDROURETRONEPHROSIS

X RAY OF
NORMAL KIDNEYS, URETERS, BLADDER

FIGURE 40   **X-RAYS**

Occasionally there is an associated malformation that allows urine to escape through a channel that connects the dome of the bladder to the umbilicus (belly button). This condition is called patent (open) urachus.

Babies with "prune belly" may also have a chest deformity. Parents must never put a binder around their baby's tummy to hold it in because this will compress the abdominal contents upward and may actually contribute to the chest wall deformity and interfere with breathing. Donald's mother wrote that she found the one-piece stretchy terry cloth suits concealed his condition better than other kinds of clothing. There are likely to be a succession of operations facing Donald and other newborn boys with this distressing defect.

Exstrophy of the Bladder. This is a deformity that results in the bladder being exposed on the outside of the body and "turned wrong-side-out."

It is not very common, occurring only once in every 30,000 live births. But, as parents remind their doctors, "Statistics are not important because, when it happens to you, it's 100%." Because it is an uncommon problem, most pediatricians want the babies transferred to a center where there is a pediatric urologist who is experienced in caring for the complex problems at hand and those to come in the future.

Since the bladder is "wrong-side-out," the ureters are exposed and the urine drips from them continuously, creating a continuous wetness problem until surgery is performed. The urethra, instead of being formed in a tube, is just a "trough." This is called *epispadias*. In boys it means that the penis is like a "trough" too and will need repair. In girls the labia are usually located higher than the usual position between the legs. Exstrophy is also accompanied by hernias, separation of the pubic bones, and the absence of a belly button because the umbilical cord is attached in the crevice where the bladder protrudes out of the open abdominal wall.

The comedian Mort Sahl used to joke about it and say that a belly button was proof that we had a mother. Thinking about it in that way, even in jest, suggests that it is an important thing to have. Marianne confided that she would never wear a two-piece bathing suit because she was embarrassed that she didn't have a belly button. Jean-Paul's mother consulted a plastic surgeon to have him create a dimple on the abdomen that would look like one. Dr. John Duckett, a pediatric urologist in Philadelphia, "made a belly button" for one of his patients "that even God would be proud of!"

It was thought for a long time that children with exstrophy would not be able to run or ride a bike because of the abnormal separation of the pubic bones. That worry was put to rest years ago. But some of the children walk with a "waddle." This may be caused as much by several layers of wet diapers as by the pelvic disorder. There may be some difference in the walk, but only enough to be noticeable to people who know about the condition. Orthopedic surgery can help.

Exstrophy in itself is not life-threatening. In fact, some urologists leave the bladder exposed until the babies are old enough to make long surgery less risky. They may perform a urostomy if they determine that the bladder is definitely too small or too deformed to ever function correctly.

Two pressing problems early in life are infection and incontinence (the inability to control urination). Urinary tract infection destroys kidney tissue. This, of course, is dangerous and parents must be alert to low-grade temperatures and other signals that infection is present.

Once the bladder has been repaired and replaced in the body, it still may not hold urine properly. Pediatric urologists have several surgical techniques they use to try to restore normalcy.

Incontinence often becomes a serious social problem when it is time for children to go to school. In fact, in the 1960s it was thought to be sufficient reason to perform a urostomy. Urologists are likely to be more conservative now, but some youngsters may not be, and some have asked for, and welcomed, an ostomy, in its place.

Sid says he's never been sorry. Tom said he was so grateful to get rid of the smelly diapers that he wished he had had the operation sooner. Susan, who lived in the cold Northeast, said the best thing about the ostomy was getting rid of the sore chapped inner thighs she used to get during the winter when she was wet all the time. After Tom's urostomy he was in a rap group that was discussing what was "normal" and "abnormal." He said, "To me dry is normal." It is important to add that some exstrophy patients finally achieve continence during puberty or late adolescence, and they are convinced it was worth waiting for.

There are later problems, too, that must be dealt with: infertility, delayed development of the scrotum, and shortening of the penis in males. And, in females there can be vaginal deformity that requires surgery before intercourse can be accomplished comfortably, and prolapse of the uterus associated with childbirth. Parents of boys and girls with exstrophy of the bladder are called upon to be brave, strong, patient, and very knowledgeable. Many, like Paul's, Richie's, and Laura's mom, have become first class nurses without an RN degree.

Spina Bifida. *Spina* refers to the spine; *bifid* means split in two. This birth defect is the most common crippler of children and afflicts two out of every 1,000 new-born infants. That means that each year about 6,000 babies will be born with spina bifida. The cause is unknown.

In its mildest form, called spina bifida occulta, nerve and motor function usually are not affected. The two forms that cause considerable damage to a number of bodily functions are *meningocele* and *meningomyelocele*.* As you look at the diagram (Figure 41), you will see that the spinal cord is intact with a meningocele. Only the covering and fluid bulge through the defect in the boney spine. But with meningomyelocele the cord as well as its covering are protruding through. In recent years an aggressive approach by a team of specialists with new medical technology has made it possible to save most of these babies.

Common problems with meningomyelocele include paralysis and loss of feeling in the legs. Many of the children will also develop hydrocephalus,** and the cerebral spinal fluid (CSF) that should circulate freely between the brain and spinal cord backs up and causes swelling of

Meninges are the covering of the spinal cord; *myelo* refers to the cord itself; *cele* means sac.
**Hydro* means water. *Cephalus* means head.

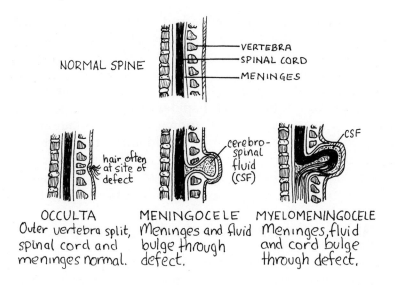

NORMAL SPINE

VERTEBRA
SPINAL CORD
MENINGES

OCCULTA
Outer vertebra split, spinal cord and meninges normal.

hair often at site of defect

MENINGOCELE
Meninges and fluid bulge through defect.

cerebro-spinal fluid (CSF)

MYELOMENINGOCELE
Meninges, fluid and cord bulge through defect.

CSF

FIGURE 41   SPINA BIFIDA

the ventricles and pressure on the brain. Fortunately, it is now possible for neurosurgeons to place tubes with safety valves that drain the fluid off the brain into another part of the body to be absorbed into the blood stream.

There are many books available from the Spina Bifida Association of America (SBAA) that explain spina bifida and its consequences in great detail. There are excellent publications by doctors and health professionals as well as some by parents. Mrs. Betty Pieper, whose son Jeff was born with spina bifida, writes from the heart of someone who has "been there." The SBAA has chapters across the country that meet together and publish regular newsletters of information for their members. In addition, the national organization holds an annual meeting. You will find the address in the resource list in Section VII.

Only rarely in spina bifida do the bladder and bowel escape damage. Sometimes the bladder won't empty and becomes a huge sac that is always infected. At other times the problem is that the bladder is small and unstable and it frequently squeezes and spurts and holds very little urine. Infection and incontinence are the usual result.

Many youngsters with spina bifida had urostomies up until about five years ago. More recently it has become possible to control both infection and incontinence with medication and the regular insertion of a clean catheter into the bladder to drain the urine. Some children will have a urostomy temporarily and then it can be closed and intermittent self-catheterization started. Before Dr. Lapides and his staff at the University of Michigan pioneered this "bold" approach, it was thought that only a sterile catheter should be used in the bladder and the strictest of sterile techniques used when inserting it. Dr. Lapides, and now many who have followed his teaching, have demonstrated that infection can be eliminated by regularly emptying the bladder before it overfills. Quite a breakthrough!*

So it may be said, in summary, that in 1981 some spina bifida children will need a urostomy, but certainly not as many as in the years past.

Bowel control is another problem that must be faced by children with spina bifida. Peristalsis in the bowel may be weak and ineffective, or spastic because of the spinal cord problem. Sometimes the children become terribly constipated and the rectum and descending colon become impacted with hard dry stool. Small but frequent amounts of soft feces make their way around, and may be mistakenly considered diarrhea. This condition is called "paradoxical diarrhea," and it is a signal to action to cleanse the colon and begin a regular anti-constipation program. Sometimes a high-fibre diet, regular toileting schedule, a daily suppository or enema, or stimulation with a gloved finger may be required to start bowel action. It is important that the children drink plenty of liquids.

There is of course a lengthly list of social reasons why bowel control is crucial. It also has been suggested by some urologists that a rectum distended (over-filled) with stool may interfere with bladder function and urination.

Seldom is it possible to achieve regular bowel habits until urinary continence has been achieved, either by catheterization or urostomy. It's a rare boy or girl who will take off wet pants to go to the toilet for a bowel movement.

One of the best things for parents of children with spina bifida is the development of the team concept for their children's care. "Birth defect clinics" or "meningomyelocele teams," that bring all the specialists together in one place, save not only wear and tear on parents and children, but also gasoline, the chore of visiting each office separately, and the

---

*Urologists vary in the technique they prefer, but one method is described in Appendix D. Mrs. Lowe, the nurse who teaches Dr. Lapides' patients, has a videotape of a six-year-old boy and girl who have become "pros" in self-catheterization. Kathleen Hannigan, a nurse at the John F. Kennedy Institute's Birth Defects Clinic in Baltimore has described in a medical journal how she taught pre-school children to catheterize themselves, using a doll as a training aid.

huge amounts of time waiting at each one. Whether concerns are neurological, orthopedic, vocational, urological, or medical, there ought to be an answer in the clinic.*

None should minimize the emotional and financial toll these children will take on their families, but neither should anyone underestimate the pride and joy that parents like Monica's and Fred's experience when their children develop into happy and productive young people in spite of their disabilities. There are those who advocate abortion, when amniocentesis (drawing out a sample of the aminotic fluid surrounding the fetus in the womb) shows the presence of alfa-fetoprotein, signalling a spina bifida baby will be delivered. A day at the annual SBAA conference will put you in touch with a legion of mothers who point with love to their children and protest against such recommendations.

Posterior Urethral Valves. It is unlikely that your neighbors have been talking about posterior urethral valves lately, but they are the most common source of urinary obstruction in infant males. Once they are suspected, the abnormal folds of tissue can be seen by a urologist's trained eye through a cystoscope (an instrument that allows visualization of the bladder and urethra). Sometimes the valves almost completely block the passage of urine, from the time the urinary tract begins to operate in the uterus, causing hydroureteronephrosis (illustrated in figure 40 with the discussion of "prune belly" syndrome). In such cases the newborn will be quite ill, and have an abdominal mass that turns out to be urinary organs swollen from dammed up urine.

There are other situations in which the obstruction is less complete, with only moderate damage. Often the babies have flu-like symptoms or simply fail to gain weight and grow like they should. This may be referred to as "failure to thrive" on the hospital chart. It may be several months or, in a few cases, several years before a correct diagnosis is made. When this occurs, parents often wish they had complained louder or looked for another, "better" doctor who "would have known what was wrong."

Urologists recognize that the symptoms rarely point to the urinary tract and urge pediatricians to be alert for such a condition in infants who run low grade fevers, have recurring gastrointestinal upsets, and who do not gain weight properly. It has proved to be a difficult diagnosis. After it has been made, the mothers have often asked why kidney X-rays aren't performed routinely to check for these deformities. It is not so simple; it would be expensive, and would subject many babies to unnecessary testing to find problems in a very few.

*In a publication from the Children's Memorial Hospital in Chicago, 20 people are listed as members of their team.

Jay's mother felt guilty for several years because the pediatrician had asked her if Jay had voided a good stream. She had answered, "yes" and told of having to wipe the wall beside the bath table when he urinated without a diaper on. She did not realize, until her second son arrived, that "a good stream" meant all the way over to the chest of drawers! Jay, in fact, had not been urinating normally.

Jay's mother, like so many other wise parents, has since learned that the bad feelings that come from "I wish I had known . . .," "Why didn't we ask?" and "If only we had . . ." are of no help at all. The sooner they can be talked out and put to rest, the better parents, family, and children will feel.

The extent of damage to the urinary system will determine whether an operation to divert the urine is needed. A urostomy may be required temporarily to permit prompt drainage of urine and to allow maximum potential recovery for the urinary tract. In some cases bladder damage is so severe that a urostomy must be a lifelong substitute (unless and hopefully until new technology produces a better solution).

Other Conditions. The foregoing are the more common childhood problems that lead to ostomies. There are others. Cancer, such as rhabdomyosarcoma, may require urostomy or colostomy or both. Some of the most deadly childhood cancers have a much more hopeful outlook now with combinations of surgery, chemotherapy, and radiation therapy.

When injury to the bowel or bladder occurs, it may be necessary to divert stool or urine away from the site of the damage to the outside of the body, to allow healing to take place without interference, or to protect surgical repair.

Injuries to the pelvis, often in motorcycle or automobile accidents, may be so severe that restoration of normal function is impossible. Paralysis of the bladder and bowel after spinal chord injury usually is handled without surgery. There may be occasions when an ostomy is indicated.

After reading this section you must be wondering how common these conditions are and how many children there are with ostomies. Perhaps you are marvelling that you've never known about ostomy until now. No one is certain how many ostomies are performed in the pediatric age group each year. One thing is for certain. Unless you live on a remote island and have little communication with the outside world, you will be amazed to begin discovering how many people—adults and children—have ostomies that you never knew about before, and how much comfort and practical information will be available from people who have "been there" already. Their support, a membership in the United Ostomy Association, and a trusting relationship with your physicians and nurses will give you the information and determination you need to successfully cope with your children's illness and treatment.

Notes

Index To Alphabetical Answers

Allergies to adhesives and skin preparations are surprisingly uncommon.

Alkaline urine harbors bacteria and should be acidified.

Antibiotics may cause diarrhea and other side effects.

Appliances for urostomies, colostomies, and ileostomies come in a wide variety of styles, colors and materials.

Asparagus gives urine a pungent odor.

Athletics need not be given up.

Belts do not keep appliances from leaking, but they do support the weight of a filling pouch.

Bleeding from the stoma is not unusual, and it isn't dangerous unless it persists or recurs frequently.

Blue bag syndrome is a harmless condition in which urostomy appliances turn navy blue to purple.

Bowel control is difficult for many children with genitourinary and gastrointestinal conditions.

Bran can be helpful as a laxative.

Changing refers to appliances.

Chemotherapy necessary to treat cancer may have unpleasant side effects.

Chicken pox doesn't spare children with ostomies and may occur under the appliance face plate.

Citrus fruits and juices are not to be confused with the Vitamin C recommended to acidify urine.

Climate affects appliance wearing time.

Clothes can be stylish without revealing the appliance.

Continent ostomies are performed infrequently in childhood.

Convalescence after ostomy operations varies according to the children's condition and the surgery required.

Convex face plates are usually recommended when a stoma is flush or the abdominal skin is soft and wrinkled.

Cost of managing an appliance may vary from under $200 to more than $500 per year.

Cushions may make sitting easier after removal of the rectum.

Danger from stomal injury is rare, but appliances can cut the stoma if they fit too snugly or if they slip.

Dehydration must be of concern for anyone who has an ileostomy.

Diet is overemphasized; most ostomates have no food restrictions.

Disability is a medical fact not to be confused with a handicap.

Dry cleaning bags make excellent mattress covers for travel.

Effluent refers to the stool or urine from an ostomy.

Encouragement is very important for child ostomates.

Encrustation occurs when skin is exposed and urine is alkaline.

Enterostomal therapists are specialists in ostomy care.

Excoriation of the skin can be treated with home remedies.

Exercise is important for ostomates, too.

Face plates are the part of the appliance that adhere to the skin.

Fat is a particular problem to ostomates.

Foam pads make a cushion between the skin and the face plate.

Gas from a colostomy or ileostomy can be kept to a minimum.

Gauze pads can be bought in bulk and need not be sterile.

Handicap refers to a limiting condition. An ostomy need not be one.

Healing after removal of the rectum may take weeks or months.

Health records should be kept up-to-date and made available to schools and camps.

Hernias can occur around the stoma.

IEP stands for the Individualized Educational Program that is required for all children in Special Education classes.

Insurance may be difficult to obtain.

Intelligence may be hard to accurately assess when children have been limited by illness.

Jogging is popular among ostomates.

Jump suits are recommended.

Keloids are outsized scars.

Love is necessary for good health.

Mainstreaming means integration into the general class in school.

Marshmallows are said to slow ileostomy function.

Mucus is normal and should not be confused with infection or pus.

Muscle tone needs careful attention after abdominal surgery.

Monilia is a fairly common fungal infection.

Night drainage is recommended for everyone who has a urostomy.

Odor associated with feces and urine is easily controlled.

Phantom pain from a limb or an organ that has been removed is a common and normal phenomenon.

Plastic sheets are recommended to protect against unexpected appliance leaks.

Play therapy teaches young children and helps them learn more about their feelings.

Pouch covers are decorative appliance accessories that minimize perspiration under an appliance.

Power of attorney gives another person permission to act in your behalf.

Quarterly magazines published by the United Ostomy Association are invaluable.

Radiation therapy may produce unpleasant side effects.

Recreation is especially good for children with disabilities.

Restrictions are few when it comes to living with an ostomy.

Rubber appliances are not as popular as they once were.

Sand can cause irritation.

Saran wrap may be used as a dressing.

Scars can require extra parental support.

Schedule appliance changes regularly!

Sections 503 and 504 of the Rehabilitation Act of 1973 protect people with disabilities from discrimination.

Six is the age when most children are able to change their appliance without assistance.

Splattering can be minimized.

Sports can be enjoyed by all ostomates.

Steroids used to treat inflammatory bowel disease may cause unwelcomed side effects.

Stones in the kidney are not uncommon among people with ileostomies and urostomies.

Substitutes for ostomy appliances and accessories require ingenuity.

Suppositories are often used to achieve bowel regularity.

Surgical suppliers are important to ostomates and should give good service.

Take ostomy supplies on airplane trips, in the car, and on outings.

Talcum powder has several uses for ostomates.

Tape used for extra security around an appliance should be chosen with care.

Travel requires preparation but need not be given up.

Underwear can be worn under or over an appliance.

UOA is the national association of ostomates.

Urinalysis and urine culture are part of the routine for urostomates.

Urinary acidifiers are recommended, to minimize infection and eliminate odor.

Vacations can be fun.

Vinegar may be recommended for cleaning urinary appliances.

Vitamin C is an effective urinary acidifier.

Vomiting leads to dehydration.

Washers, in ostomy parlance, refer to circles of karaya or pectin wafers.

Water is not harmful to a stoma, and is needed for drinking.

Wicks made of cotton or gauze are helpful when changing a urostomy appliance.

Wipe stool and urine from appliance spouts to prevent unnecessary odors.

X-rays are commonplace. but should not become too common.

Yellow, but only pale yellow, is the color of dilute, uninfected urine.

You, the mothers and fathers of ostomates, are powerful forces in your child's growth and development.

Youth groups for young ostomates have been organized in several sections of the country.

Zephiran chloride is an effective urinary disinfectant for appliances.

Zinc oxide may be recommended when no appliance is worn.

Alphabetical Answers to Most Frequently Asked Questions

OSTOMY SPOKEN HERE was a bumper sticker that appeared several years ago. A review of this section will suggest that there is "a whole new language" to be learned with your child's ostomy. In a very short time you will speak it fluently, and the highlights included here will be "old hat" to you.

Space has been provided in the back of the book for your notes and questions. Also, please note the sincere request on p. 168 for your contributions to other parents. Anything from A to Z will be considered for inclusion in future printings.

Allergies to adhesives and skin preparations are surprisingly uncommon. Skin irritation occurs more often from scrubbing skin too vigorously with soaps or solvents, cements, etc., or failing to allow products to dry according to manufacturers' differing directions; and seepage of stool or urine under the face plate.

Alkaline urine has a pH of greater than 6.5. You can measure pH easily be allowing a drop or two of urine to run over Nitrazine paper that can be purchased at the drug store. (If you apply the Nitrazine paper directly to the stoma, you will get an incorrect reading because the stomal mucosa is alkaline.) A high fluid intake is recommended, to maintain dilute, uninfected, acid urine.

The most common causes of alkaline urine are infection, insufficient fluid intake, and dirty reusable appliances. No matter what precautions are taken, stagnant urine becomes alkaline as bacteria multiply. Urine that collects over several hours, or during the night in an appliance, will be alkaline and will have a foul odor. This urine can cause stomal inflammation, stenosis, encrustation and painful granulation on surrounding skin. Wash reusable appliances with vinegar-water solution, zephiran chloride, or an ostomy appliance disinfectant. Use night drainage to keep alkaline urine away from the stoma.

Prescription for alkaline urine: Force fluids, unless another condition prohibits it; drink cranberry juice; reduce intake of citrus fruits and juices to a minimum (4 oz. per day); experiment with an acid-ash diet if necessary (See Appendix C); take urinary acidifiers as prescribed. If, after following these suggestions, alkaline urine persists, look for infection.

A urine specimen should be collected by catheterizing the stoma using sterile technique. NEVER COLLECT OR ALLOW TO BE COL-

LECTED ANY SPECIMEN FROM THE APPLIANCE FOR URINALYSIS OR CULTURE!

Antibiotics may be necessary to treat an infection, but they may cause diarrhea or contribute to skin reactions.

Appliances come in assorted shapes, sizes, colors, and materials. Many adults with a protruding stoma, located on a flat abdominal mound, find it more convenient to wear expendable appliances, that are worn for several days (up to seven) and thrown away. Children, on the other hand, often need to change their appliance every two or three days; and reusable appliances are more economical and may provide more security against leakage.

Asparagus causes urine to have a pungent odor within hours after it is eaten. It is often recommended that people with urostomies avoid it for this reason. As long as the pouch is odorproof there seems to be little reason to pass this vegetable by if it's a favored food.

Athletics are an important part of growing up. They should not be given up because of an ostomy. Physicians often advise their patients against participating in contact sports to avoid injury to the stoma—or kidneys when there has been previous damage to the urinary tract. In truth, children with ostomies have participated in all sports, even football, karate, weightlifting, and wrestling, which often top the "forbidden" list. However, it is important to understand the risks as well as the possible benefits. And it is imperative that the coach and the school be informed of the ostomy.

Belts do not prevent appliances from leaking. They do support the weight of a filling pouch. Many adults do not wear belts. Most children, who may not be as careful about emptying their appliance, do wear them. Belts should not be clinched tightly because they could do harm to skin, internal organs and even promote a hernia. Some elastic stretches enormously when it gets wet. After swimming, a bath, or a shower, a dry replacement will be needed. Rubber belts are often recommended for swimming and bathing. Belts last longer when they are not put in the dryer; they should be washed frequently to maintain their fresh smell and appearance. A soft comfortable mesh elastic belt is sold by several suppliers, including the Parthenon Company.

Bleeding from the stoma is not unusual. If it persists more than an hour, if it does not stop when ice is placed over the stoma, or if the stoma is swollen or has changed color, consult your physician. Don't panic—a few drops of blood in a pouch full of urine may look like a hemorrhage!

Blue bag syndrome is an unusual phenomenon in which urine from a urostomy turns appliances, drainage tubing, etc., navy blue to deep purple. The urine itself is normal in color, occasionally dark yellow.

Most children whose urine has discolored all their appliances have had two things in common: their urine has been infected and it has had a pungent, repelling odor. While these two symptoms are problems in themselves, blue bag syndrome is a benign condition.

Bowel control has been difficult for many children. Those with spina bifida have problems because of neural damage and lack of sensation. Children who have had pull through operations and ileorectal anastamoses after removal of their colon have been troubled with frequent loose stools and perianal excoriation. Skin care must be meticulous.

Some encouraging preliminary reports on the successful use of biofeedback in establishing bowel control have been reported by Dr. Marvin Schuster and his colleagues of the Baltimore Maryland City Hospitals.

Bran is recommended as an effective laxative and is thought to be good for many things "that ail you"—from obesity to diverticulosis! Pure bran, a natural food fiber, is available at health food stores and some large grocery stores.

Children are not always delighted by the taste. Sometimes you can get them to eat 2-3 tablespoons mixed with peanut butter and jelly for a fatter sandwich. Sometimes you can add that amount to oatmeal while it is cooking.

With thanks to the sources, here are two excellent recipes for bran muffins.

BRAN RAISIN MUFFINS

1	cup all purpose flour	½	cup raisins
1	tsp. baking power	1	egg (beaten)
½	tsp. baking soda	⅓	cup molasses
½	tsp. salt	¾	cup milk
1½	cups bran	2	Tbsp. *melted* shortening

Stir flour, baking powder, soda, and salt. Stir in bran and raisins. Moisten with combined egg, molasses, milk and shortening. Stir until thoroughly blended and bake in greased muffin tins at 400° for 20 to 25 minutes.

From—*By, For and With Young Adults with Spina Bifida* by Betty Pieper, Spina Bifida Association of America

OLLIE's BRAN MUFFINS

2	6-oz undiluted frozen orange juice	2	eggs
		½	cup butter
2	mashed bananas (1 jar "Junior Food" bananas may be substituted)	4	cups All Bran cereal (or,
		1½	cups pure bran and 2½ cups All Bran)
1	cup flour	1	cup raisins
2	Tbsp. baking soda		

Mix thawed orange juice and bananas. In a large bowl mix flour, baking soda, eggs, butter, bran. Add orange juice/bananas mixture and raisins. Fill greased pans to top (the batter does not rise). Bake at 375° about 20 to 25 minutes.

From—*Side Exit,* Santa Barbara Chapter, United Ostomy Association

Changing an appliance refers to taking one off and putting on another. It does not mean switching from Brand X to Brand Y.

Chemotherapy necessary in cancer treatment may make children quite ill and cause them to have frequent loose stools. Ostomy care may be more difficult during these treatments, but usually parents have a number of supportive people available to help promote the children's comfort.

Chicken pox and ostomies are a poor combination but they do occur. And the pox will form under the appliance face plate. It is important to use a skin barrier that is not difficult to remove and not irritating, in itself, to the sores.

Citrus fruits and juices are excellent sources of potassium and Vitamin C. However, the Vitamin C in citrus fruits is NOT to be substituted for the ascorbic acid or natural vitamin C tablets (that might be prescribed for urostomies) because citrus fruits and juices actually are metabolized into alkaline urine.

Climate affects wearing time of appliances. It may be necessary to change appliances more often when the temperature is hot and humid. Skin barriers tend to disintegrate more rapidly in southern climates. Take this into consideration when packing for a vacation.

Clothes make the man! And the boys and girls. Normal clothing should be no problem for children who have ostomies except for their associated conditions. Bathing suits may require more attention before purchase. Black and navy blue show moisture LESS than lighter colors, where incontinence is a problem. Flowers and bold prints make it nearly impossible to find an appliance outline.

Continent ostomies have been and are being performed. (A continent colostomy, using a magnet implanted under the skin around the stoma, with a cap of the opposite magnetic pole, was developed in Germany. Several hundred of these operations have been performed on adults in Europe, and some in the United States. The results have gotten "mixed reviews.") This is not an operation for children.

The continent ileostomy was discussed briefly on p. 23. Though its success rate has continued to improve, and complications are being reduced, young children probably will continue to have conventional ileostomies. They can have them converted to a Kock pouch (see p. 23) if they are suitable candidates, when they get old enough to care for it reliably. At the present time it must be said that nearly all urostomies require an external appliance.*

Convalescence varies from child to child, ostomy to ostomy. Some children are still shuffling down the hall, stooped and pale, at the end of two weeks. Others have been chafing to return to school. Speak with your physicians whenever you think that events are not occurring on schedule. Do not risk becoming upset by erroneous assumptions or expectations.

Convex face plates are available with most models of reusable appliances. This curvature against the body often makes a more effective seal when the stoma is flush, the abdominal skin is fleshy and wrinkled, or the stoma is situated in a crease or a fold. (Figure 42)

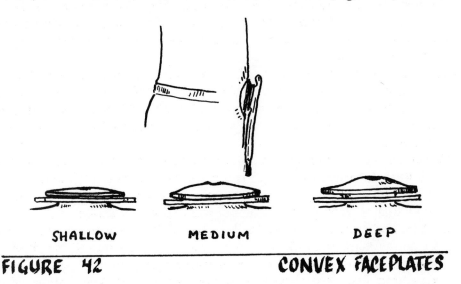

SHALLOW   MEDIUM   DEEP

FIGURE 42   CONVEX FACEPLATES

Cost of managing an ostomy varies greatly. In 1981 some people are getting by on as little as $175-$200.00 per year. The cost of managing children's ostomies is usually more because they change their appliances more frequently. Financial assistance may be obtained through some private insurance companies, Medicare, Medicaid, and Crippled Children's Services in your state. Many military hospitals are able to furnish appliances for military dependents.

Cushions are comfort items recommended in the first days and weeks after removal of the rectum. The popular donut-shaped cushion is

*A continent urostomy has been Professor Nils Kock's goal for a number of years. Dr. Alex Gerber in Alhambra, California, who spent some time with Dr. Kock in Sweden, has performed two such operations in the U.S. Mr. Michael Handley-Ashken of Norwich, England, has reported on his attempts to accomplish an appliance-free urostomy.

NOT recommended because when patients sit on them, their buttocks are actually pulled apart, making the discomfort worse. A thick square foam cushion is preferable.

Danger! During the summer when children are swimming and perspiring, their appliances may slip enough to cut into the stoma but not enough for the slippage to be noticed. Bleeding from the stoma or swelling should be investigated immediately. A cut in the stoma may heal by itself if a larger face plate is used temporarily. The edges of the stomal opening in expendable appliances (such as Coloplast Stoma Urine) may become very sharp after they have been wet for a day or two. (Figure 43) It is advisable to protect the peristomal skin with a skin barrier and allow at least ⅛" between the base of the stoma and these appliance openings to reduce the possibility of stomal laceration.

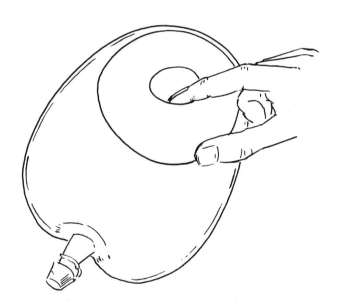

FIGURE 43   EDGE MAY BECOME SHARP

Dehydration must be a concern for anyone who has an ileostomy because the colon, which normally absorbs fluid, is absent. According to doctors specializing in sports medicine, thirst is not a good indicator of dehydration—it comes AFTER you have become dehydrated. Unless there is a coexistent medical condition that contradicts the general rule, children with ostomies should learn early to drink plenty of fluids frequently—4 to 6 glasses per day.

Diet is frequently overemphasized. Few children with ostomies require a special diet. Sensible nutrition and good eating habits should be encouraged in every family. It is important that children with ileostomies and colostomies be taught to chew their food well. More detailed diet information is offered in Appendices A, B, C.

Disability is an emotional word. No one wants to admit to one. Less than 20/20 vision is a disability that can be corrected with glasses. Ostomies are disabilities that may be managed with appliances. Disability is not synonymous with handicap!

Dry cleaning bags make excellent mattress covers when visiting because they're easy to come by and easy to pack. Take enough so you can throw them away when you move on to the next stop.

Effluent refers to what comes out of the stoma. Ileostomy effluent changes according to diet and length of time since eating. Colostomy effluent is also affected by food and fluid intake. It is common to see recognizable remnants of a meal, such as a tomato skin, in an ileostomy pouch. Because the effluent from fecal ostomies is thicker than from urostomies, the appliance openings are slightly larger and the outlet spouts are larger too.

Encouragement is something that all children need. Children with ostomies need it more! Encourage them to develop hobbies, encourage talents, encourage self-care and self-reliance. Encourage a healthy body image and positive self-esteem.

Encrustation is a condition commonly found on skin surrounding children's urostomies. (Figure 44) When you see encrustation, there probably is some degree of stomal stenosis (narrowing—see Glossary). Dirty gritty urinary appliances with accumulated urinary calcification should be discarded. The affected skin should be covered with a skin barrier. It may be treated in the doctor's office with a silver nitrate stick. Fluids should be forced and night drainage should be used.

Residual urine in the conduit indicates stomal stenosis, and calls for more vigorous treatment. Remove the appliance daily and apply acetic

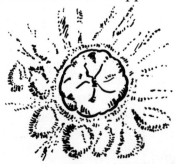

FIGURE 44   **ENCRUSTATION**

acid soaks for 30 minutes, using 1 part white vinegar to 3 parts water. Saturate a gauze pad with this solution and place it over the stoma and affected skin. Remove after 5 minutes and replace with a freshly saturated gauze pad; 6 fresh pads should be used during the treatment. At bedtime put 2 ounces of the vinegar/water mixture in the bottom of the appliance. Instruct the child to lie down and let the mixture bathe the stoma for 10-15 minutes.

Enterostomal Therapists (ETs) originally were lay people, either with ostomies or who had children with ostomies. These ETs, as they were called by the late Dr. Rupert Turnbull of the Cleveland Clinic, were more than a group with a good idea who started charging a fee for helping people with appliance problems. They were interested, knowledgeable, and concerned people who had been identified by surgeons and INVITED to come into hospitals to assist the medical staff and teach the nurses.

The first meeting of enterostomal therapists was held in 1968. The International Association for Enterostomal Therapy was formed officially, under another name, in 1969. There are 1135 members of the Association. As it should be, ETs are now required to first be registered nurses before taking the training.

Excoriation (red, raw skin—see Glossary) usually has a simple remedy, even when the skin is raw and bleeding. Wash the affected area gently with mild soap and water. Rinse and pat to dry. Cover with Stomahesive and an appliance. (Think of the Stomahesive now as a bandage or dressing.) Remove in 48–72 hours unless there is evidence that urine or feces has leaked under the Stomahesive. You should see dramatic improvement in 2–3 days. Continue until skin is well-healed. Consult an ET or a physician if marked improvement in comfort and appearance is not achieved in 48 hours. IT IS NOT NECESSARY—AND IT IS ILL ADVISED—TO PUT ANY MEDICATION, OINTMENT OR GLUE BETWEEN DAMAGED SKIN AND STOMAHESIVE!

Exercise is important at every age. Passive exercise, massage, active and programmed exercise—all have their place. Exercise is essential for good health. Seek guidance from your physician or physical therapist to insure that your child gets sufficient and appropriate exercise.

Face plates must fit correctly—both outside and inside diameter. The stomal opening should be about ⅛" larger than the stoma for a colostomy or ileostomy and only 1/16" larger than a urostomy stoma, unless it is the throw-away type discussed above. The outer edges should not cut in or cause abrasions. Most reusable face plates can be easily customized with a Dremel Tool or a less expensive reproduction from J.C. Penney's. (Figure 45)

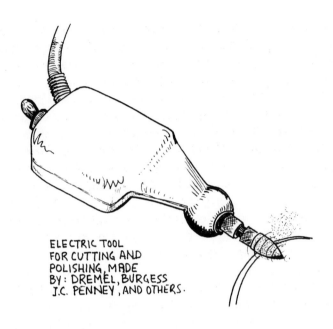

ELECTRIC TOOL
FOR CUTTING AND
POLISHING, MADE
BY: DREMEL, BURGESS
J.C. PENNEY, AND OTHERS.

FIGURE 45

Fat and ostomies make a hopeless combination. Fat is unattractive; fat is unhealthy; fat makes it difficult to wear an appliance. Many parents believe, often in the depths of their subconscious, that fat means insurance against illness and signifies recovery and a good outcome. Nothing could be farther from the truth.

Foam pads used to be recommended frequently to provide a cushion between a rigid face plate and the skin. They are not used as much nowadays, because fewer reusable appliances are used. But they are still a valuable accessory to know about. They are a part of the Nu-Hope expendable appliance systems. It is important that the foam pad be CLOSED CELL; that is, the foam will not absorb liquid. If your child is wearing a foam pad, and a rash or irritation that exactly corresponds to the pad develops, look to absorption as the problem.

Gas (flatus) is a common concern. Sometimes antacids will reduce gas. Chewing food well and with the mouth closed will minimize the problem. Gas is the product of swallowed air, bacterial action, and chemical processes in the intestine. A pouch with an outlet for flatus should have a closure or a charcoal filter so that odor is not constantly seeping out. (See the discussion of diet in Appendix A)

Gauze pads are excellent wipers and blotters. They may be bought in bulk, and may be covered by your insurance if they are a necessary part of ostomy care. There is no reason to purchase sterile, individually packaged gauze pads for the majority of ostomies.

Handicap is a condition that interferes with normal or necessary activities. An ostomy need not be a handicap unless, of course, your child aspires to be a belly dancer. However, attitudes about ostomy may be handicapping. Watch out for them. Appliances that leak frequently are severely handicapping. If your child has such a problem, consult an enterostomal therapist or an experienced surgical supplier at once.

Healing of the perineal wound after removal of the rectum may take months. Pads will be required for wound drainage. Those with adhesive strips to keep them in place in undergarments are a convenience. There are many variables that must be considered when projecting the time required: the type of closure, the patient's nutritional state, whether the patient has been on steroids for a long period of time, etc. Each surgeon has his own method of care for the perineal wound, which will take into account the patient and the type of surgery performed.

Health records are important to your child. In most cases they get very thick. It is a good idea to have a summary updated every couple of years. If you keep six or seven copies of the summary at home, you will have one on hand for schools, camps, travel, and a visit to a new physician.

Hernias can occur at the site of the stoma because the opening in the abdominal wall made for the stoma interrupts the abdominal musculature. Heavy lifting and weight lifting probably should be avoided. (The kitchen garbage is not considered heavy lifting! Neither are most grocery sacks!)

IEP stands for Individualized Educational Program and it refers to the assessment and planning required for children who qualify for special education in public schools. If your child requires "Special Ed," YOU play an important role in the development of the IEP.

Insurance and insurability may be compromised by an ostomy. Occasionally the problem stems from an uninformed insurance clerk. More often there are REAL problems. On the other hand, you may qualify for more insurance benefits than you realize. Consult the surgical supplier from whom you purchase your child's appliances and accessories; consult the company through which you have health insurance; if you want life insurance, you may have to shop around. The social service department of the hospital, and the United Ostomy Association may be able to furnish important information.

Parents of one young man with an ostomy and severe kidney disease, who had tried unsuccessfully for years to purchase insurance for him in spite of his apparent good health, were delighted to receive a solicitation by mail that offered insurance to college-age youngsters for a small annual payment: "No medical questions asked; guarantee to purchase larger amounts at age 25." They could hardly get it in the mail fast enough after they had checked to see that the company was reputable.

Intelligence is far more than a score on an IQ test. Children who have had frequent hospitalizations, and operations that challenged their physical and mental stamina, frequently have more "savvy" than average children. At the same time, visual motor perception, measurable knowledge, skills, and acquired information may have suffered from lack of stimulation, inactivity, or anesthesia. Parents need to work with school teachers, counselors, and psychologists in order to get an ACCURATE assessment of their child's aptitude and potential.

Learning disabilities are not uncommon among children who have ostomies. It is scary when they are incorrectly labelled "slow" or "retarded" and are not taught ways to compensate. Whether you think your child has a learning problem, is "just average," or is gifted, you are that child's best advocate. And do keep in mind that intelligence can be cultivated and exercised.

Jogging is a current fad. Even when the fad passes, many will continue to jog because they have found that they look better and feel better. There are many jogging members—young and old—of the United Ostomy Association. Pouches should be emptied, of course, before the run begins.

Jump suits are marvelous garments for infants and toddlers with ostomies, because they cover the ostomy and the pouch and keep small hands from pulling on the bottom of the pouch or playing with the contents.

Keloids are outsized scars that may cause trouble for a person with an ostomy, particularly if the scar will be underneath a face plate. If your child forms keloids, bring this to the surgeon's attention, and at the same time point out scars on other parts of the body.

Love is surely as necessary to life as food, fresh air, and a heart beat. Children who are or have been sick need large doses of love laced with high expectations and firm discipline. Parents who have sacrificed for children with demanding health needs require love and reassurance too. Look for it, plan for it, and provide it.

Mainstreaming is the term used when discussing the integration into public schools of children who earlier would have been in "special schools." Children with an ostomy, without other disabilities, should have no problems in public schools. Mainstreaming is discussed in more detail on p. 62.

Marshmallows have been recommended by ileostomates as handy items to have on hand to slow the ileostomy flow when changing an appliance. No, the marshmallow is NOT inserted in the stoma! It is said that if you eat one or two marshmallows 15 to 20 minutes before you change your appliance, the stoma will be less active. It's worth a try for children who like marshmallows anyway, and who need their appliance changed at a time of day when their ileostomy normally is quite active.

Mucus threads are a normal part of the urinary output from an ileal or colonic conduit because the intestinal segment secretes mucus. If they clog the outlet valve, there are products such as Mucosperse® (Marlen) available to dissolve them in the appliance before emptying. A mucous fistula (see Glossary) may secrete so much mucus that a gauze pad or dressing must be worn over it.

Muscle tone needs attention after abdominal surgery. After the surgeon has given the "go ahead," calisthenics or aerobics may be helpful in tightening abdominal and other sagging muscles.

Monilia is a fungul infection that may appear on the skin. It is characterized by a localized, red irritated rash around the ostomy. It will respond quickly to the application of an anti-fungul powder, such as Mycostatin®, and topical anti-inflammatory spray, such as Kenalog® or Decaspray®. Consult an ET or your physician if you suspect that your child's skin reaction is a monilial infection.

Night drainage is probably the most resented but most necessary part of urostomy care, particularly for children. For spending the night out or

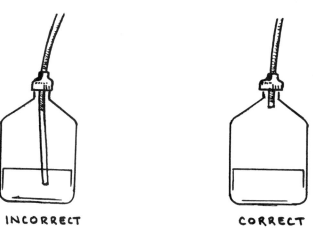

INCORRECT   CORRECT

FIGURE 46   **NIGHT DRAINAGE**

camping trips, a leg bag is easier and less conspicuous than a night drainage bottle. The world will not come to an end if it is not used on an occasional night out, but the risk of an overflowing pouch that leaks on a friend's bed or in a sleeping bag must be considered.

Appliance manufacturers sell a variety of bedside connections. It is not difficult to make one from a long piece of tubing and a bleach or empty vegetable oil container. TAKE NOTE: IF THE LEVEL OF URINE RISES ABOVE THE END OF THE TUBE, DRAINAGE WILL CEASE AND A VACUUM WILL OCCUR. (Figure 46)

Odor is a natural part of bowel movements but it is dreaded by ostomates, young and old. There are preparations that may be taken by mouth, drops that can be put into the appliance, solutions that are used to wash pouches, and room sprays and powders too. All are listed and available from well-stocked surgical suppliers. You will do well to remember three creeds:

—Dilute, uninfected urine does not have a foul odor.

—Everyone's bowel movements have an odor, some more offensive than others.

—Never create, with store-bought deodorizers, odors more offensive than those you are trying to mask!

Phantom Pain or sensations that they need to have a bowel movement are not uncommon among children and adults who have had their rectum removed. Sometimes sitz baths help. These pains have been likened to those experienced by amputees when feet that are no longer there itch.

PL 94-142 is a Federal law that affects all children with disabilities between the ages of 3 and 21. It is discussed in more detail on p. 142.

Plastic sheets are a good idea to protect the mattress when appliances leak, but children should never be made to sleep next to the plastic. There are contoured plastic sheets and also the type that encases the whole mattress and zips closed.

Play therapy may be a formal program, conducted in or out of the hospital by health professionals, or it may be parents' creative contributions to their children's discovery and learning. Help your children grow and accommodate to their ostomy by using play as a means of therapy.

Pouch covers are made of cotton, jersey, or other soft fabrics. They minimize perspiration between the appliance and the skin. They are not just a luxury item that only the vain should wear, though they do also look nice. They are easy to make at home, or they may be bought from Foxy Enterprises,* in a variety of patterns, colors, and shapes and coordinated with other undergarments.

*See p. 151, Ostomy Appliances and Incontinence Aids.

Power of attorney gives a relative or babysitter the authority to consent to medical treatments of minors in the absence of their parents. If you need to be away and are giving someone responsibility for caring for your child, check with the hospital to see what their rules are. Normally a power of attorney can be drawn up simply by writing a statement: "We, the parents of Tom Smith, give Mrs. Sam Brown authority to consent to any medical treatment our son requires during our absence." Once the statement is signed (and usually also notarized), it becomes an effective legal document, and a safeguard to your child's health.

Quarterly is how frequently the United Ostomy Association publishes its invaluable magazine, *The Ostomy Quarterly*. All the latest appliances and accessories are introduced in this publication. There are wonderful stories by and about those who have had ostomies and the successful adjustment they have made; and there are helpful hints about all kinds of ostomies and related conditions. The journal plans to start a column especially for parents. If you do not subscribe now, you are missing an essential resource. Write to the United Ostomy Association, 2001 W. Beverly Blvd., Los Angeles, CA 90057.

Radiation Therapy (x-ray treatments) for cancer may cause skin changes that interfere with appliance wear. They also may require modification of the appliance or application procedure during the course of treatment. Enterostomal therapists (particularly those who have had experience with ostomates who have required radiation therapy) can be most helpful in offering solutions that will keep the children as comfortable as possible.

Recreation is good for everyone; it is especially good for children with disabilities. Hobbies, sports, music, collections, etc., may all be a source of entertainment and a means of developing a positive self-concept.

Restrictions? Perhaps the greatest concern of parents, and the most frequent misconception among health professionals as well as lay people. There really are not ANY universal or absolute restrictions limiting children with ostomies. Some parents will unnecessarily restrict activities and social experiences thinking that they will protect their children from physical or emotional injuries. Some will modify their diet because they find the stool easier to manage. None should *ever* restrict fluid intake to reduce the frequency of appliance emptying.

Maybe there's a cynical reader who would say, "Aha, they certainly can't go to a nude beach!" But the Los Angeles UOA chapter's newsletter recounted the story of a brave ostomate, who had always wanted to experience a nude beach and finally ventured out—camera over the shoulder and ostomy pouch in place. A passerby commented, "That's a handy way to carry your film."

Rubber appliances and tubing are considered by many to be passé because they tend to retain odor, require time-consuming cleaning, and are bulky. There still are many ostomates, mature and young, who are wearing them. Black butyl rubber is amazing in its non-odor-retaining properties.

Sand from the ocean beach or sandbox may get underneath an appliance belt and cause irritation (without producing a pearl). It's a good idea to remove your child's belt after trips to the beach or the sandbox, and to put on a fresh one after washing the skin.

Saran can be used to cover an infant's exposed bladder or intestinal mucosa if a pouch is not to be worn. The Saran will prevent the mucosa from drying out and protect it from irritation by a diaper.

Scars are often embarrassing to children. At various stages of their development they will flaunt them (like President Johnson once did on national television), and at other times they will wear an unsightly T-shirt over a bathing suit to cover a mark that makes them different. Some say cocoa butter or vitamin E oil on scars will help them become less noticeable. The value of these remedies is questionable; but just doing SOMETHING to the scar, perhaps by putting cocoa butter or vitamin E on it may make youngsters feel better! There are cosmetic cover-ups too. Parents are encouraged to be supportive.

Schedule appliance changes. Do not wait for leakage. Planning a time and place for this, even if it's every day or every other morning, reduces the incidence of embarrassing leakage that children will have to deal with. It further reinforces the fact that their ostomies are a part of them that requires regular attention, like brushing teeth. It is best to change urinary appliances in the morning before the children have anything to drink, when the urinary flow is considerably less. Ileostomies usually are easier to deal with before meals or several hours after eating than they are an hour or two after taking food. Of course, when leakage does occur, appliances should be changed as soon as possible. But why is it that it usually happens five minutes before the guests are due, or ten minutes after, or just after you've put the chicken in to fry?

Sections 503 and 504 of the Rehabilitation Act of 1973 are important to anyone with a disability who is seeking or will seek employment. The specifics of this law are discussed on p. 142. Local public employment offices will have even more detailed information.

Six is generally the age when children are able to take off and put on appliances without assistance. Some can do it earlier, some need another year or so to mature. It requires hand-eye coordination and spatial perception that simply may not be present until six to eight years of age. Children, no matter how hard their mothers try, are not likely to keep their hygienic standards up to par. They will need help and supervision.

It is a good idea for fathers to help their sons as the boys get older. This is likely to foster a closer father-son relationship, and it also will reinforce the boy's masculinity and remove the embarrassment caused by a mother's intrusion on bodily privacy.

Splattering when an ileostomy appliance is emptied in the toilet may cause an unsightly and offensive mess at home or at friends'. Adults with ileostomies have said that it is helpful to pull the flush handle just as they open the tail spout. This reduces the splash when the fecal contents are emptied into the water.

Sports contribute to the development of an effective body image and positive self-esteem. They are an important part of growing up during middle childhood and adolescence, as much for girls nowadays as for boys. When children are too small, too frail, or simply unable to participate in team sports, it is wise to encourage them toward sports or other activities in which they can test their limits and savor their accomplishments. There are many fulfilling activities besides sports that nurture body and spirit (collections, hobbies, playing musical instruments, etc.)

Steroids such as cortisone often are used to treat inflammatory bowel disease. They may produce an array of unpleasant side effects: weight gain and puffiness, mood swings, and impaired wound healing, among others. They also may control the disease! When children have been on cortisone prior to surgery, it is customary to reduce their dosage afterward. Gradually they taper down on dosage before going off completely.

Stones in the kidney are not uncommon among people with ileostomies and urostomies. In fact, they are high on the list of possible complications. Sometimes they pass spontaneously, without surgery; other times an operation is required to remove them. Guarding against dehydration by drinking plenty of fluids is one way to minimize the risk of kidney stones.

Substitutes for forgotten or lost ostomy supplies are not easy to come by, but there are a few. Fingernail polish remover may be used to remove adhesive residue. Wash the skin thoroughly afterwards! Shoe laces are EXCELLENT substitutes for "O"-rings that secure a pouch to a face plate. Rubber bands will do too. Rubber bands, paper clips, and clips from the stationery store may be used as appliance closures.

If you are away from home you probably will have the most success by looking under "Surgical Supplier" in the yellow pages for an advertiser that sells ostomy appliances, or calling a member of the Ostomy Association in that city. A list of chapters and contacts is published regularly in the Ostomy Quarterly—as handy to have as a map when you're traveling.

The best thing is to have a check list, plan ahead, never allow yourself to run low, and DOUBLE CHECK before you leave on a trip!

Suppositories often are used as a part of a bowel regimen, particularly for children with spina bifida who have a neurogenic bowel. It may be difficult for them to retain the suppository. It has been recommended that the buttocks be taped together or that the children or their parents hold them in place until they have dissolved.

Surgical suppliers might be likened to grocers. There are good ones and bad ones. There are small, intimate ones where your minimum purchase is treated as their privilege and you are a friend; and there are large impersonal ones with a vast selection and special "deals." There are all sorts in between. You may want the security of being able to stop in for your purchases at a neighborhood pharmacy or ostomy dealer. You may be delighted to pick up the phone or fill out an order blank to a supplier in a distant city.

A few generalizations can be made: Prices are competitive on today's market and you may be able to save money by shopping around. You do not, and probably should not, do business with a dealer who is frequently "out" of what you need. An occasional back-order may occur; but when it happens several times, you can find improved service elsewhere. There are surgical suppliers who keep records of everything your children use and all the sizes; there are suppliers who fill out Medicare and Medicaid forms; there are those with informative newsletters; and there are some who custom-cut Colly-Seels and Stomahesive to the dimensions of the face plate. There is even one who includes jelly beans for the children in most shipments! If you are not CONSCIOUSLY APPRECIATIVE of your surgical supplier, you probably need a better one.

Take ostomy supplies with you on the airplane. Do not put them with your luggage. When you go to Miami and they go to Memphis, that is misery for you and your child! And take an ample supply for the length of time you will be gone. Take a change of appliance and change of clothes even on short day trips. It is a simple precaution that will increase your child's physical and psychological comfort should unexpected leakage occur. ALWAYS TAKE A CHANGE OF APPLIANCE AND INSTRUCTIONS WITH YOU TO THE HOSPITAL, X-RAY DEPARTMENT AND PHYSICIAN'S OFFICE.

Talcum powder and babies go together like bread and butter. It also is a useful addition to ostomy care. Talcum powder sprinkled lightly inside reusable appliances, before they're hung to dry, keeps them from sticking together (except when Stomahesive is used). Talcum powder underneath the pouch may help minimize perspiration and guard against heat rash in hot weather. Cornstarch on the skin is soothing. Non-greasy talcs are preferable to highly scented powders with additives.

Tape is probably used by everyone with an ostomy at one time or another. Two tapes which are preferred by many ostomates come to the U.S. from England: Chironplast® (by Downs) and Hy-Tape® (distributed by Byram, Bruce, Kay's and others). Both are pink. They are waterproof, slightly elastic, and as harmless as any to sensitive skin. Consult your surgical supplier. There are also several good paper tapes, such as Scanpor® (Bard Home Health) and Micropore® (3M). Do not use old-fashioned adhesive tape. Do NOT use any tape that irritates your child's skin.

Travel need not be a problem for children with ostomies. In fact, for a boy named Jimmy it was much easier after an ostomy. He had been incontinent of urine and his mother had had to take a suitcase full of clothes and diapers. The older he got the bigger the suitcase his mother had to pack, until finally she quit the annual trip to grandmother's. Eight weeks after Jimmy's urostomy she called to thank her ET and describe what fun they had had traveling again, and how easy it was with just his few ostomy supplies.

For youngsters with inflammatory bowel disease there should be similar freedom—freedom to travel farther and farther from the toilet to which so many have had to cling.

Travel of any length requires preparation. It is good to have a check list and to designate one responsible person to put the appliances and necessaries in the car or travel bag. Theoretically, it should be the child's responsibility; but children have been known to forget. Double check.

There are several helpful names to know when traveling internationally. The International Ostomy Association is an organization of national ostomy associations in 32 countries around the world. The address of contacts in the countries you plan to visit may be obtained from the UOA office in Los Angeles.

The International Association for Medical Assistance to Travelers (IAMAT), 350 Fifth Avenue, Suite 5620, New York, NY 10001 has a directory for its members with the names of English-speaking physicians in hundreds of cities in 120 or so countries. Membership is free. You do not have to have an ostomy to know that this sounds like a comforting membership to have! Their Canadian office is at 1268 St. Clair Ave. W., Toronto, Ont., Canada M6E 1B9.

Medic Alert Foundation International, Department AZ, PO Box 1009, Turlock, CA 95380 is the non-profit organization mentioned earlier that provides an emergency medical identification system that can be tapped from anyplace in the world. Theirs is the organization with the distinctive necklace or bracelet that alerts helpers to a special medical condition.

For traveling with all the information one should have for a safe and enjoyable trip, there is no better book than *Access to the World* by Louise Weiss. Written as a travel guide for the handicapped, it is a treasure for everyone. After all, who among us is immune to diarrhea or sprained ankles in foreign lands? If you do not see this book at your local bookstore, you can write Louise Weiss at 154 E. 29th St., New York, NY 10016. The cost is under $10.00.

Traveling is a part of learning, growing, and enjoying life. Ostomies and related disabilities should not interfere.

Underwear may be worn under or over an appliance. Most children are happiest when their appliance is tucked into panties or jockey shorts. It does not harm the stoma if the elastic waistband lies over the appliance. The Atlantic Surgical Co. in Merrick, New York, advertises a sportsman's and sportswoman's undergarment. They do not list a pediatric size, but such a brief might be nice for a bigger child. Whatever the garment, whatever the age of the wearer, it is important that any elastic be loose enough to permit two fingers to slip easily underneath, that it not be so tight that urine or stool cannot pass from the stoma into the appliance, and that it be kept meticulously clean. Nylon underpanties with a cotton crotch, or cotton pants are recommended for girls.

UOA is the national association of more than 600 chapters and 42,000 people who have ostomies or are interested in their care. The United Ostomy Association had its beginnings in a Veteran's Hospital in Philadelphia in 1949. In the next few years it became clear that the people who knew most about ostomy care, even when they didn't know much, were ostomates themselves.

The UOA had its official Constitution Convention in 1962. Their symbol is the Phoenix Bird; their standard, "Reborn from the ashes of disease." UOA has an annual conference each August where more than 1,000 people gather for educational and social meetings.

UOA should take credit for increasing public awareness; contributing to professional education; stimulating manufacturers to improve ostomy appliances and accessories; and, through their volunteer visitor program, lifting the spirits of thousands of terrified people, who thought they couldn't go on with an ostomy.

A frightened young mother remembers her letter to the Philadelphia Chapter in 1963. No, they did not have any information about children with ostomies, but they were concerned. They understood. And this was more help than anyone else had ever been. A beautiful young woman remembers her despair as a teenager at the thought of having an ostomy—until a UOA visitor of nearly the same age came to call. There are countless similar stories of encouragement and assistance.

The dues are low; the rewards are high. Whether you only read the magazine (that comes every three months) or become an active participant in local and national programs, you will find that the United Ostomy Association has more information about living with ostomies than any other source. Write to them at 2001 W. Beverly Blvd., Los Angeles CA 90057.

Urinalysis and urine cultures from urostomies should be obtained from the stoma, using a sterile catheter and sterile technique. DO NOT ALLOW A SAMPLE OF URINE TAKEN FROM A UROSTOMY POUCH TO BE USED FOR URINALYSIS OR CULTURE.

Urinary acidifiers may be recommended to acidify your child's urine. Cranberry juice is an excellent acidifier if consumed in large quantities. A little is probably better than none at all. Most children must acquire a taste for it. Cranberry juice can be fattening and may be purchased with artificial sweeteners. Vitamin C (ascorbic acid) is an effective acidifier when taken in sufficient amounts. Even small children may require 250 mg. four times a day to keep the pH of their urine below the advisable limit of 6.5. There are prescription medications too, but the most important prescription for children, to keep their urine acid is, "DRINK PLENTY OF LIQUIDS."

Vacations are supposed to be fun. But vacations without ostomy supplies and necessary prescriptions are no fun for anyone. PLAN AHEAD.

The opportunity for parents to take a vacation away from their children is often pushed aside by parents of children with medical conditions. They, more than most, probably would benefit from the respite and relaxation. Older children with ostomies say they are thrilled with every chance they get to "be on their own." Whether you are planning a vacation with your children or leaving them at home, be systematic in your preparations.

Vinegar is frequently recommended for cleaning urostomy appliances. White vinegar is better than cider vinegar, only because it is colorless. A vinegar-water solution (1 part white vinegar to 3 parts water) will disinfect appliances and night drainage bottles; it is best to insert it into the bottom of the appliance to bathe the stoma when there is stomal inflammation caused by alkaline urine; and it is a good soak for encrustations of the peristomal skin. It may be made up in large quantities, using non-sterile water. Rinse everything well. Otherwise the person or the product will smell annoyingly like a salad bowl.

Vitamin C (ascorbic acid) has been mentioned several times as an effective urinary acidifier. It is available in chewable tablets for small children.

Vomiting leads to dehydration in a very short time. Whether it is caused by the flu or an obstruction, children who are vomiting should probably be seen by a physician. Gatorade and similar drinks are excellent sources of electrolyte replacement after strenuous exercise or gastrointestinal upsets that lead to fluid loss.

Washers, in a discussion about ostomies, are neither machines that do laundry nor little round black things that stop faucets from leaking. Washers refer to wafers of karaya, karaya amalgams, or synthetic tacky substances that serve as barriers to irritation caused by stool, urine, or adhesives on the skin. Many companies sell washers in a variety of sizes. Many people cut their own. If you have a small child and you are using 2½"–3" Stomahesive or Hollihesive washers, you will save money by purchasing the 8" × 8" sheets—even if they do seem much more expensive at the outset.

Water is necessary to live. It is particularly necessary for children with ostomies. Offer glasses of water frequently.

Water is also fun to swim in and swimming is a wonderful sport that can be enjoyed by even the most severely disabled. Children with ostomies who swim a lot may need to change their appliances more often, even if they use waterproof tape to "picture frame" the face plate edges. But that should not be a deterrent to fun and good exercise. (Belly flops from the diving board are discouraged!) Appliances should be worn in pools, oceans, and lakes. They need not be worn in bathtubs or showers. Water will not hurt a stoma.

Water that is not clean may cause illness if consumed. If you are traveling in regions where water treatment is questionable, bottled water may be a sensible precaution for everyone in the family (a matter of particular concern for ostomates).

Wicks to absorb the constantly dribbling urine from a urostomy stoma are helpful, when changing the appliance. They may be made by rolling one nonsterile gauze square into a cylinder and holding the end to the stoma. No need to mash. Tampons make excellent wicks, but they never should be offered to boys unless all reference to their traditional use is removed. Many parents use the corner of a wash rag or towel and then throw it in the day's laundry. Rolled toilet tissue will also do. Cotton is usually a mess.

Some youngsters with urostomies report that it is helpful to "bend over and touch their toes a few times" before beginning to prepare their skin for an appliance application. This, they say, seems to "milk" the urine out of the conduit.

Wipe—teach them to wipe! Failure to wipe stool from the tail closure of an ileostomy or colostomy pouch, or urine from the outlet valve will cause soiling of the clothes and offensive odor—odor that surely will cause teasing from playmates.

X-rays are commonplace for children with ostomies. There are barium enemas, IVPs, etc., etc. Children who are subjected to frequent x-rays of the abdominal region should have their gonads (ovaries and testes) covered with a lead apron or drape. Further, if you are seeing several doctors who are ordering x-rays, or you move frequently and new physicians request x-rays, STOP! Sit down with one physician and review the amount of x-ray your child has had, the x-rays that are essential to the preservation of good health, and the most sensible way to avoid overexposure. Be certain, too, that your child's films are in a safe repository so they are not lost or misfiled.

Yellow, pale yellow to nearly colorless, is the color of dilute uninfected urine. If your child's urine is thick, and dark gold in color, increase fluids. Suspect infection if there is a foul odor. Some stool softeners cause urine to turn orange. Pyridium, which is a urinary antiseptic, also causes urine to turn a bright orange. There are also preparations that may be swallowed to color the urine blue when the doctor is looking for a fistula.

You, as mothers and fathers, are powerful forces in the growth and development of your children. They need love; they need limits; and they need advocates. You, more than all medical and surgical expertise, will determine the kind of life your children experience as young people and the future they make for themselves as adults.

Youth groups for young people with ostomies are functioning in several cities. The United Ostomy Association has sponsored two Youth Rallies. The first was in Denver, CO in 1978, and the second was in Chevy Chase, MD in 1979.

The young people who attended were excited by the opportunity to "rap" with their peers who REALLY understood. Many stayed up through the night. For some it was a first opportunity to meet someone who had had the same operation. Even though he had been told repeatedly that "many children have this operation," one little boy was absolutely thrilled when he SAW that his roommate had an ostomy too!

There are youth activities scheduled at the UOA annual conferences and chapters are encouraged to plan activities for young people. There is an ad hoc committee within UOA to assess the needs of parents of children with ostomies. There have been proposals to have a column set aside in the Ostomy Quarterly for issues and concerns specific to youth and in which youth can share their successes.

Even though they may not want to have frequent meetings, children can get worlds of information from others their own age. Carol was typical of many busy teens when she said to her mother, "You told me that I would be 'normal' after this operation and now you want me to go to these meetings to be reminded once a month that I'm abnormal. I don't want to go to any meetings, but I'll be happy to call some kids or go see them when they need surgery or after they've had it." On the other hand, some young people have served in the Ostomy Association as they might in scouting or other volunteer activities. They have been contributors to their chapters and leaders in youth groups. Your children will let you know what's right for them.

Zephiran chloride is a disinfectant that can be purchased at the drugstore without a prescription, to clean urostomy appliances and accessories. With a prescription, it probably will be covered by your insurance.

Zinc oxide is commonly recommended for use around babies' colostomy stomas when an appliance is not going to be used. Remember that ointments of any kind should not be used with appliances because they interfere with the adhesive seal. If zinc oxide is being used, please take care to remove it completely at least once a day. Some terrible skin irritations have occurred under zinc oxide and other cream applications that were repeatedly layered, allowing stool to seep and get trapped next to the skin.

Resources That Help

Nearly everything you would ever want or need to know with respect to disabilities generally can be found in *The Source Book for the Disabled* (p. 148). The resources listed here are those that will be particularly helpful for parents of young ostomates.

First, it is necessary to come to grips with the words that may be used to describe your children—"disabled" and "handicapped." A disability is a medically determined fact that can be described and defined. A handicap is any limitation. An analogy serves to make the distinction. The figure skating champion Dorothy Hamill has a disability. She does not have 20/20 vision, and must wear glasses. Actually she has been able to capitalize on her disability by advertising eyeglasses and making money from it. Had she wanted to enter pilot training in the Air Force, she would not have qualified, and would have discovered that her disability was a handicap.

Children with ostomies have a disability, a medically determined fact that can be described. In order that they not become socially, academically, vocationally, or financially handicapped, you are encouraged to take advantage of any or all of the following resources.

Financial Assistance

STATE

Medicaid is a state administered program that provides specified coverage for medical care and equipment. Entitlement is based upon family income. The hospital social service department will have information. You also may write to the Department of Human Services, Washington, D.C. 20201, for a free pamphlet, "Medicaid—How Your State Helps When Illness Strikes," that explains the difference between Medicaid and Medicare.

Crippled Children's Service uses a combination of state and federal funds that usually are administered through the county or state. The hospital social service department should have information. Your children do not need to be crippled, in the common usage of the word, to qualify for assistance.

FEDERAL

Medicare and Social Security administer insurance and supplemental funds for people with disabilities. The hospital social service department may be helpful to you in obtaining and interpreting information.

Know what medical items and services are deductible at income tax time. Write United Cerebral Palsy Association, 66 E. 34th Street, New York, New York, 10016. (They have a good booklet.)

The Law

Sections 503 and 504 of the 1973 Rehabilitation Act pertain to non-discrimination and affirmative action.

Section 503 stipulates that every employer doing business with the Federal Government under a contract for more than $2,500 must take "affirmative action" to hire handicapped people. Affirmative action covers more than hiring. It also covers job assignments, promotions, training, transfers, working conditions, terminations, etc.

Section 504 stipulates that every institution in the United States getting Federal financial assistance must take steps to assure that handicapped people are not discriminated against in employment. Included are schools, colleges, hospitals, nursing homes, social service agencies, and many more kinds of institutions and establishments.*

PL 94-142 is the Education For All Handicapped Children Act of 1975. It requires "free, appropriate public education" to all handicapped children ages 3 through 21. Part of the law requires that an IEP, individualized education program, be formulated for each child. The IEP is required to have specific goals and to be reviewed regularly. Parents participate in the development of their children's IEP. Another key phrase in this legislation is "least restrictive environment." These three words are the ones that keep children who do not need to be in schools for the severely disabled, in classrooms with children whose disabilities are less severe, or in regular classrooms with time out for remedial classes.

Within organizations such as the Spina Bifida Association there is further information about specific legal issues and rights. If you still have questions, write or call:

*From "Affirmative Action for Disabled People—a Pocket Guide," for sale by the Superintendent of Documents, U.S. Government Printing Office, Washington, D.C. 20402.

National Center for Law and the Handicapped
1235 N. Eddy Street
South Bend, IN 46617
(219) 288-4751

Information, Education and Psychosocial Support

The UNITED OSTOMY ASSOCIATION has given parents hope when there was none, direction when there was nothing but confusion, and an opportunity to reach out to others along the way. The UOA has more than 600 chapters in cities across the United States and in Canada. Besides the excellent *Ostomy Quarterly* they publish every three months, each chapter has a newsletter and the Association has a long list of books, monographs, and films. Membership dues are minimal and the return on your money, even if you were never to attend a meeting, would far exceed your investment. Write today to the
United Ostomy Association
2001 W. Beverly Blvd.
Los Angeles, CA 90057
(213) 413-5510

The SPINA BIFIDA ASSOCIATION OF AMERICA, like the UOA, has a national headquarters that serves as a clearinghouse and administrative office for chapters across the United States. If your child has spina bifida, this is the first call you should make, the first letter you should write:
Spina Bifida Association of America
343 S. Dearborn—Suite 319
Chicago, Illinois 60604
(312) 663-1562

The ASSOCIATION FOR THE CARE OF CHILDREN'S HEALTH, is a multidisciplinary association promoting the psychosocial wellbeing of children and families in health care settings. Its members include health professionals, parents, educators, and a wide variety of specialists concerned with education and advocacy to promote children's health.
The Association for the Care of Children's Health
3615 Wisconsin Avenue, N.W.
Washington, D.C. 20016
(202) 244-1801

The AMERICAN CANCER SOCIETY has an extensive ostomy rehabilitation program and you need not have cancer to benefit.
American Cancer Society, Inc.
777 Third Avenue
New York, NY 10017
(212) 371-2900

The AMERICAN SOCIETY FOR PSYCHOPROPHYLAXIS IN OBSTETRICS is dedicated to the Lamaze approach to childbirth and to better, more informed parenting. In addition to prenatal classes, ASPO sponsors postpartum discussion groups for new mothers and their babies. They have an extensive recommended reading list.
American Society for Psychoprophylaxis in Obstetrics
1411 K Street, N.W., Suite 200
Washington, D.C. 20005

The INTERNATIONAL CHILDBIRTH EDUCATION ASSOCIATION is an interdisciplinary organization representing groups and individuals, both parent and professional, who share a genuine interest in family centered maternity care. The ICEA bookcenter reviews and sells books on a variety of subjects from childbirth, to child care, to parent care.
International Childbirth Education Association
PO Box 20048
Minneapolis, MN 55420

CLOSER LOOK is a clearinghouse for information pertaining to children with disabilities.
Closer Look
PO Box 1492
Washington, D.C. 20013

National Easter Seal Society for Crippled Children and Adults
2023 Ogden Avenue
Chicago, IL 60612

National Foundation for Ileitis and Colitis
295 Madison Avenue
New York, NY 10017
(212) 685-3440

National Foundation /March of Dimes
1275 Mamaroneck Avenue
White Plains, NY 10605

American Association for Health, Physical Education and Recreation
  Programs for the Handicapped
1201 16th Street, N.W.
Washington, D.C. 20036

The UNITED CANCER COUNCIL is coordinator of independent cancer
agencies throughout the United States.
  United Cancer Council, Inc.
  1803 N. Meridian, Rm 202
  Indianapolis, IN 46202

The INTERNATIONAL ASSOCIATION FOR ENTEROSTOMAL
THERAPY is the organization of nearly 1200 enterostomal therapists
(ETs) who are especially trained to care for people with a stoma and other
draining wounds and associated problems. To locate an ET closest to you
or to obtain information about the organization's activities and publica-
tions, write:
  IAET
  505 North Tustin
  Suite 219
  Santa Ana, CA 92705

And, finally, there are international organizations for ostomates and enterostomal therapists. For information regarding the International Ostomy Association, you may write the UOA. Direct requests for information about the WORLD COUNCIL OF ENTEROSTOMAL THERAPISTS
to:
  WCET
  Norma N. Gill, ET
  c/o Worldwide Ostomy Center, Inc.
  926 E. Tallmadge Ave., Suite C
  Akron, Ohio 44310

Betty Pieper, who is a prolific author for the Spina Bifida Association,
suggests that parents keep lots of post cards handy to write various
associations and agencies, and companies that look like they might have
something to offer. Maybe they won't, but just maybe they will have
something very important that you need.

  Other sources of help may be found in your community. Look under
"Social Services" in the yellow pages to see what listings are there that
could be useful to you. If you think your child needs home health care or
home teaching, a few telephone calls will put you in touch with the
appropriate people. For home nursing there is usually a Visiting Nurses

office and private agencies. ("Social Services" or "Nurses and Nurses Registries" in the Yellow Pages). The amount of coverage provided by your insurance depends upon the insurance plan and whether you have a physician's prescription. Your local schools or hospitals should be able to give you details on home tutoring.

Many hospitals have parent support groups. Some meet during the day. Others are held in the evening so more fathers can attend. If they are available, do not miss them. It is helpful to share with others who are experiencing similar feelings and situations. Sometimes it's a great comfort to see for yourself that you are not doing "nearly so bad" in comparison to others. There are few parents, even if they protest that they don't need it or "didn't learn anything I didn't already know," who leave a parent support group without more insight than they came in with.

If you should have to take your child to a distant medical center for hospitalization, there are Ronald McDonald Houses in several cities, and more being completed all the time, where parents can stay close to their children for a nominal fee. (This has been a major project of the McDonald's Hamburger Corporation.) Check with the hospital to which you are going or the one from which you are being sent for information; or write: "Bud" Jones, Golin Harris Communications, 500 N. Michigan Ave., Chicago, IL 60601.

Books to Read

FOR CHILDREN

Tommy and His Stoma by Ellen Shipes, RN, MN, ET
    Tommy had to have an ostomy. He was taught to take care of it, but he did not do so well after he returned home. A visit back to the clinic caused him to improve his care and the story has a happy ending. A delightful coloring book for children. Available from International Urological Sciences, PO Box 408, Long Valley, NJ 07853. (201) 852-8789.

All About Jimmy by Carol Norris, Ph.D.
    A coloring book that explains to children the various ostomies and why they might be performed. The drawings are delightful and the story line excellent. Available from the United Ostomy Association, 2001 W. Beverly Blvd., Los Angeles, CA 90057. (213) 413-5510.

The Sneetches and Other Stories by Dr. Seuss
    One group of Sneetches has stars on their bellies. They think they are superior to the Sneetches who have none. In the end they'll all find out

it doesn't matter. OUTSTANDING story for children with ostomies to stimulate a discussion about their ostomy and about attitudes toward other differences. Random House, 1961.

A Teenager's Ostomy Guide by Bonnie Bolinger, RN, ET
From interviews and experience with others who have had this type of surgery. Written by an ET who is the mother of a young woman with an ostomy, this booklet is short and pithy and speaks to teenagers in sensitive and sensible language about the subjects most on their mind. Available from Hollister, Inc., 2000 Hollister Dr., Libertyville, IL 60048.

Shotzie's Spina Bifida Rules
A cheerful and informative six-page booklet of health rules for children with spina bifida. Available from the Spina Bifida Association of America, 343 South Dearborn St., Suite 319, Chicago, IL 60604. (312) 663-1562.

By, For and With Young Adults With Spina Bifida by Betty Pieper
Information and counsel from the mother of a young man with spina bifida. Available from Spina Bifida Association of America, 343 South Dearborn St., Suite 319, Chicago, IL 60604. (312) 663-1562.

Where Did I Come From? by Peter Mayle
The facts of life without any nonsense and with illustrations—the most wonderful illustrations you can imagine. Dr. Spock says, "I give this book top grades for humanness and honesty. Some parents will find that its humorousness helps them over the embarrassment. Others may be offended." See for yourself. An outstanding book for all children. Lyle Stuart, 1973.

What's Happening To Me? by Peter Mayle
A guide to puberty from the authors of "Where Did I Come From?" Just as good as their first. It's a toss up whether the information or the illustrations are the most delightful. Lyle Stuart, Inc., 120 Enterprise Ave., Secaucus, NJ 07094, 1975.

FOR PARENTS

The Ostomy Book by Barbara Dorr Mullen and Kerry Anne McGinn, RN
A wonderful book that explains ostomies of all kinds and ostomy-related information in a sensitive and readable fashion. Barbara Mullen had a colostomy. Kerry McGinn is her daughter. Bull Publishing Co., P.O. Box 208, Palo Alto, CA 94302. (415) 322-2855.

The Physical and Psychosocial Care of Children With Stomas by Sharlene Jackerson Hutchinson, RN, MS and Ellen A. Shipes, RN, MN, ET

Topics include basic anatomy, emotional impact, pouching procedures and equipment needs, school preparation and related subjects. Charles C. Thomas, Springfield, IL 1981.

Living With Surgery by Paul J. Melluzzo, MD and Eleanor Nealon
A book that describes the before and after effects of big operations like ostomies, mastectomies, and amputations and discusses the impact of such birth defects as spina bifida and cleft palate. A wonderfully human and straightforward volume. Lorenz Press, 501 E. Third St., Dayton, OH 45401.

The Source Book for the Disabled edited by Glorya Hale
". . . an up-to-date reference work that offers helpful and realistic advice on all the practical aspects of daily living." So say the publishers. Readers will find everything from sex to clothing modifications to addresses of agencies and organizations. A fabulous compendium of information. Paddington Press, 95 Madison Ave., New York, NY 10016, 1979.

FOR PROFESSIONALS

Principles of Ostomy Care edited by Debra C. Broadwell and Bettie S. Jackson.
Finally a definitive text that includes up-to-the-minute principles and practices of care of people with stomas and draining wounds. Whether the reader is looking for specific anatomical and physiological facts or psychosocial and sexual implications, all can be found in this 815-page compendium that will benefit every discipline within the health care team. The C. V. Mosby Co., 11830 Westline Drive, St. Louis, MO 63141. 800-345-8501. 1982.

FROM UOA

Colostomies—A guide
Ileostomy—A guide
Urinary Ostomies—A guidebook for patients
My Child Has An Ostomy
Sex, Courtship and the Single Ostomate
Sex, Pregnancy and the Female Ostomate
Sex and the Male Ostomate
Introductory Brochures
Reprints of articles about children and families and how they coped with ostomy.
Ostomy Quarterly
The Ostomy Library

FROM SBAA

Straight Talk—Parent to Parent
When Something is Wrong with Your Baby: Looking in and Reaching Out
The Teacher and the Child with Spina Bifida
Beyond the Family and the Institution: Residential Issues for Today
By, For and With . . . A Discussion for Young Adults with Spina Bifida

ADDITIONAL SOURCES OF BOOKS TO READ:

The U.S. Government Printing Office
Washington, D.C. 20402

Human Policy Press
P.O. Box 127
University Station
Syracuse, NY 13210

MAGAZINES

The Exceptional Parent (Bi-Monthly)
P.O. Box 641
Room 708 Statler Office Building
20 Providence St
Boston, MA 02116

Accent on Living
PO Box 700
Bloomington, IL 61701

The Ostomy Quarterly (Quarterly)
United Ostomy Association
2001 W. Beverly Blvd.
Los Angeles, CA 90057

Children's Health Care (Quarterly)
Association for the Care of
Children's Health
3615 Wisconsin Ave., N.W.
Washington, D.C. 20016

Pipeline (Bi-monthly)
Spina Bifida Association of America
343 S. Dearborn, Suite 319
Chicago, IL 60604

Bookmarks (Twice yearly)
International Childbirth Education
Association
PO Box 20048
Minneapolis, MN 55420

A selected bibliography follows in Section X. Classics such as Virginia Satir's *Peoplemaking* and Dr. Lee Salk's *What Every Child Would Like His Parents to Know* are referenced there.

Publications such as *The Ostomy Quarterly* and *The Source Book for the Disabled* will provide more information than you know what to do with—at one reading. But just knowing where to find it will be helpful later.

Parents are reminded never to underestimate or underrate the value and power of their own personal resources. The helper-therapy principle has generated research to show that people who are in the role of helpers gain as much as their helpees. Many books, such as Betty Rollin's *First You Cry*, are the product of personal restoration and rehabilitation. Betty Pieper, the Spina Bifida Association's versatile mother-teacher-author and Board Member, wrote:

By reaching out to others, helping with a newsletter or starting a pilot parent program, for example, one starts to work through his or her own feelings and to find meaning in what happened to him. It is one of life's greatest satisfactions to be handy with the right kind of information at the right time and to thus ease someone else's way.

Perhaps you, too, will find comfort and new coping energy from becoming active—say, in the United Ostomy Association or in the school or hospital volunteer corps.

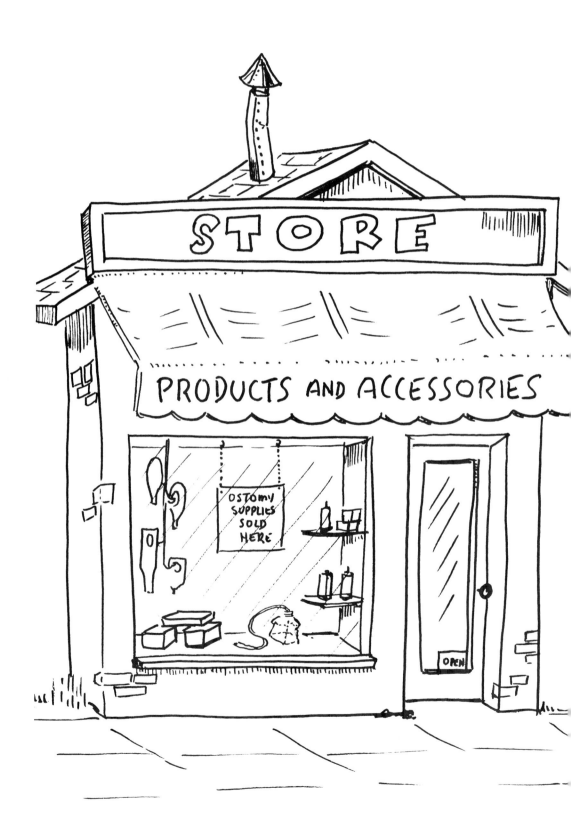

Ostomy Appliances and Incontinence Aids

For a Listing of Dealers in Your Area Consult The Ostomy Quarterly and the Yellow Pages of Your Telephone Directors Under "Surgical Supplier"

Atlantic Surgical Company, Inc.
1834 Lansdowne Avenue
Merrick, New York 11566
(516) 868-4545

B & R Ostomy Specialists
2432 S. Colorado Blvd.
Denver, Colorado 80222
303-758-5874

Bard Home Health Division
(Manufacturer and distributor of
Coloplast, Davol, and Diamond Shamrock ostomy appliances.)
C. R. Bard, Inc.
Berkeley Heights, N.J. 07922

Berkeley Medical Supply, Inc.
2041 Center St.
Berkeley, CA 94704
415-848-1023

Blanchard Ostomy Products
2216 Chevy Oaks Road
Glendale, California 91206

Bruce Medical Supply
411 Waverly Oaks Road
Waltham, Massachusetts 02154
800-225-8446
In Massachusetts: 800-342-8955

Byram Surgical, Inc.*
2 Armonk Street
Byram, Connecticut 10573
(203) 531-6400
In New York: (212) 829-5320

Convatec, a division of
E. R. Squibb and Sons, Inc.
P. O. Box 4000
Squibb Hospital Division
Princeton, New Jersey 08540
(609) 921-4000

Cornwells Pharmacy
317 E. 39th Street
Vancouver, WA 98663
206-694-1548

Crescent City Pharmaceut.
1509 Tulane Ave.
New Orleans LA 70112
504-524-2254

Custom Service, Inc.
220 71st Street, Suite 214
Miami Beach, Florida 33141
(305) 861-3666, 3667

D'Odor Corporation
3400 Forsyth Road
Orlando, Florida 32807
(305) 671-7508

Dynamed Corporation
200 Clearbrook Rd.
Elmsford, N.Y. 10523
(914) 592-5430

Fogelson Pharmacy
100 W. Osburn Road
Phoenix, Arizona 85013
602-274-3635

Foxy Enterprises
Plaza 16
E. Lancaster Avenue
Ardmore, Pennsylvania 19003
(215) 642-6207

Gatti Medical Supply
1231 York Road
Abington, PA 19001
215-338-9200

John F. Greer Company, A Corp.
530 East 12th Street
Oakland, California 94606
(415) 465-4162

Hollister, Inc.
2000 Hollister Dr.
Libertyville, IL 60048
(312) 680-1000

Kay's Ostomy Center*
4085 Tweedy Boulevard
South Gate, CA 90280
(213) 564-1745
(714) 994-2761

Kelley Ross
511 Olive Way
Seattle, Washington 98101
206-622-3565

King & Moore
4515 Brainard Rd.
Chattanooga, Tenn. 37411
615-698-8586

Knueppels Pharmacy
8405 W. Lisbon Ave.
Milwaukee, Wisconsin 53222
414-462-0550

Marlen Manufacturing and Development Co.
5150 Richmond Road
Bedford, Ohio 44146
(216) 292-7060

Mason Laboratories, Inc. (Colly-
Seels)
P. O. Box 334
Horsham, Pennsylvania 19044
(215) 675-6044

Medical West Pharmacy
950 Francis Place
Clayton, Missouri 63105
314-725-1888

Mentor Corporation*
1499 West River Rd. North
Minneapolis, MN 55411
(612) 588-4685

Miami Ostomy Center
8051 Northeast 2nd Ave.
Miami, FLA 33138
305-759-5043

Miller's Inc. Home Health Svcs.
139 Forrest Ave. N.E.
Atlanta, Georgia 30308
404-659-4300

Nova
POB-45 Route 28
Centerville, Mass. 02632

Nu-Hope Laboratories
2900 Rowena Avenue
Los Angeles, CA 90039
(213) 666-5249, 5248

Osto Care Company
P. O. Box 2131
Sepulveda, CA 91343

The Parthenon Co., Inc.
3311 West 2400 South
Salt Lake City, Utah 84119

The Perma-Type Co., Inc.
P. O. Box 448
Farmington, CT 06032
(203) 677-7388

Prescription Center
  915 Hay Street
  Fayetteville, N.C. 28305
  919-484-6214

Rystan Company, Inc.
  470 Mamaroneck Avenue
  White Plains, New York 10605

St. Louis Ostomy and Medical
    Supply
  11722 Manchester Road
  St. Louis, MO. 63131
  (314) 821-7355

Shelton's Pharmacy/Medical Sup-
    ply
  1525 Wayne Avenue
  Dayton, Ohio 45410
  (513) 253-4108
  (513) 294-0232

Shield Health Care Center
  6705 Val Jean Ave.
  Van Nuys, CA 91406
  213-786-1935

Stein Medical
  3724 W. Wisconsin Avenue
  Milwaukee, Wisconsin 53208
  (414) 342-7755

Suburban Health Services
  430 S. Main St.
  N. Syracuse, NY 13212
  315-458-1231

Suburban Ostomy
  214 N. Main St.
  Natick, Mass. 01760
  800-225-4792

Sween Corporation
  P. O. Box 3404
  Mankato, Minnesota 56001

Torbot Company, Inc.
  1185 Jefferson Boulevard
  Warwick, Rhode Island 02886
  (401) 739-2241

United Division of Howmedica
  11775 Starkey Road
  Largo, Florida 33540
  (813) 392-1261

Vance Products, Inc.
  1100 W. Morgan Street
  P.O. Box 227
  Spencer, Indiana 47460-0227
  800-457-4422

Worldwide Ostomy Center
  926 E. Tallmadge Ave. Ste. C
  Akron, Ohio 44310
  216-633-0366

*These companies specialize in incontinence as well as ostomy products.

SKIN CARE PRODUCTS

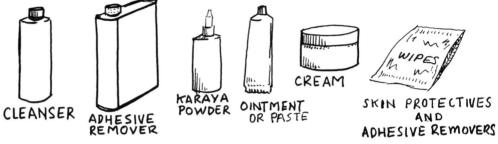

CLEANSER   ADHESIVE REMOVER   KARAYA POWDER   OINTMENT OR PASTE   CREAM   SKIN PROTECTIVES AND ADHESIVE REMOVERS

SKIN BARRIERS

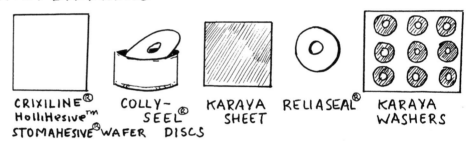

CRIXILINE® HolliHesive™ STOMAHESIVE® WAFER   COLLY-SEEL® DISCS   KARAYA SHEET   RELIASEAL®   KARAYA WASHERS

APPLIANCES
ONE PIECE EXPENDABLE (THROW AWAY)

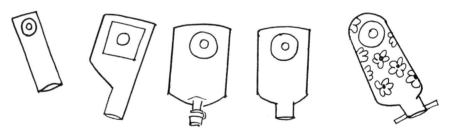

TWO PIECE EXPENDABLE (THROW AWAY)

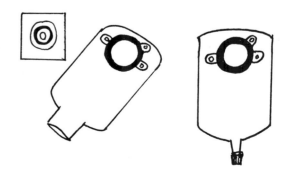

APPLIANCES

TWO PIECE (REUSABLE FACEPLATE, POUCH DISCARDED AFTER SEVERAL WEARINGS)

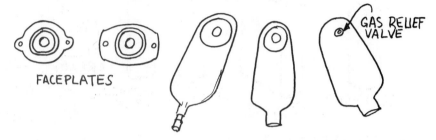

FACEPLATES

GAS RELIEF VALVE

ONE PIECE REUSABLE (VINYL OR RUBBER)

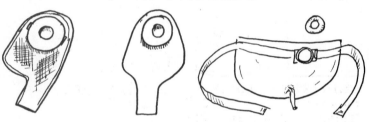

ACCESSORIES

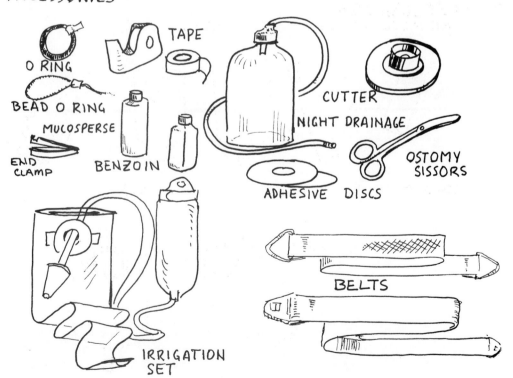

O RING

TAPE

BEAD O RING

MUCOSPERSE

CUTTER

NIGHT DRAINAGE

END CLAMP

BENZOIN

ADHESIVE DISCS

OSTOMY SISSORS

IRRIGATION SET

BELTS

DEODORANTS

BISMUTH
SUBGALLATE
TABLETS, TAKEN
BY MOUTH

TABLETS
FOR THE
POUCH

PARSLEY,
TO BE
EATEN

DROPS
FOR THE
POUCH

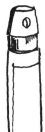

ODOR
ANTAGONIST
SPRAY

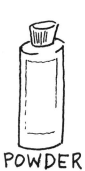

POWDER

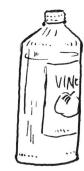

WHITE
VINEGAR

NOTES

OSTOMY   Until recently a suffix. Now (at least among involved professionals, patients and caretakers), an accepted word used to discuss the various surgically created openings into the gastrointestinal or urinary sy

PE

PE
u

glos.sa.ry   (glos'ə rē)   ten

PERISTALSIS   A squeezing rythmic motion found in the alimentary canal and the ureters in the urinary tract.

pH   Indicator of acidity or alkalinity—frequently used in discussion of urinary pH. Uninfected urine usually is on the acid side of neutral. Bacteria do not grow   thrive in alkaline urine. Patients with urina   dication, diet, or advice to drink cranbe

for

POSTERIOR   In back

PROCTOSCOPY   Visua   by means of a hollow instrument, a proctoscope.

PROJECTILE VOMITING   The forceful ejection of vomit, distinguishable from s   ith minor upsets. Vomit is also re

PROLAPSE   A   **young**   omy nomenclature, prolapse i   e bowel through the stoma.

PROSTHESIS   An artificial device used to replace a missing limb or body part.

PROXIMAL   Nearest th   origin. Opposite of distal.

PURULENT   Consist   **and**

REFLUX   A flowing b   e bladder back up to the kidney is abnorma.

REGIONAL ENTERITIS   See ileitis.

RESECTION   Surgical removal or excision.

RESIDUAL URINE   U   or intestinal conduit. This is an undesirab'   **old**   f urine invites bacterial overgrowth and

RETRACTION   The ac   omas retract into the body making management very difficult.

REVISION   Surgical relocation of the stoma to a new site or reconstruction of the stoma at the present site.

SIGMOIDOSCOPY   Visual examination of the rectum and lower part of sigmoid colon with a sigmoidoscope.

SKIN BARRIER   The term commonly used to describe synthetic gelatin-

Glossary

The following definitions are given in the context of ostomies and related conditions.

ABDOMINOPERINEAL RESECTION   An operation in which the sigmoid colon, rectum, and anus are removed. The end of the remaining colon is brought out on the abdominal wall to form a permanent colostomy.

ABSCESS   A collection of pus resulting from the disintegration of tissues.

ADHESIONS   Internal growth of scar tissue following surgical cutting. Adhesions may cause abnormal binding of parts and obstruction in organs such as the intestines.

ADHESIVE DISC   Thin paper or cloth disc with adhesive on both sides used to adhere ostomy appliances to the body. (Also referred to as double-backed or double-faced adhesive; in England it is called double-sided plaster.)

ALIMENTARY CANAL   Tubular structure consisting of the mouth, esophagus, stomach, small intestine, large intestine, rectum, and anus.

AMNIOCENTESIS   A test of the amniotic fluid that will reveal the presence of certain abnormalities of an unborn baby. A needle is inserted through the abdominal wall into the womb to draw out a sample of fluid.

ANASTAMOSIS   The surgical joining together of two or more hollow organs. When ostomies are discussed, an anastamosis may refer to the rejoining of an organ after a segment has been removed or the placement of one into another.

APPLIANCE   The pouch or device worn over a stoma to collect urine or stool. There are two kinds of appliances: single-use or expendable (sometimes referred to as "temporary" or "post-op"), and reusable (sometimes erroneously described as "permanent").

BAG   A container for groceries, lunches, and garbage. A word that most people wish were not used to describe ostomy appliances and pouches.

BARIUM   A white chalklike substance that enables visualization of the digestive tract on x-ray.

BENIGN   Not cancerous.

BIOPSY   Removal of a small piece of tissue from the living body for microscopic examination.

BUN Blood urea nitrogen. A rough index of kidney function is provided by measuring the urea nitrogen level in the blood. Normal levels are 8-18 mg %.

CARCINOMA Cancer; malignant growth.

CECOSTOMY The surgical opening of the cecum. It usually is a temporary procedure to rest the colon.

COLITIS Inflammation of the colon.

COLON The large intestine, which begins in the right abdomen and extends from the cecum to the rectum.

COLONIC CONDUIT The term used to describe a form of urinary diversion in which one or both ureters are tunnelled into an isolated segment of colon that functions as a conduit for the urine to the outside of the body. (See Figure 22)

COLONOSCOPY Visual examination of the colon made possible by the use of a colonoscope, a snake-like tubular instrument that is inserted in the anus and can be threaded through the entire length of the colon to the cecum.

COLOSTOMY Surgical opening into the colon. (See Figures 2, 3, 4)

CONGENITAL Present or existing at the time of birth, e.g., a deformity, disease, or tendancy.

CREATNINE A substance excreted by the kidney, the measurement of which indicates kidney function. Creatnine may be measured by taking a specimen of blood. The normal range is 0.5-1.0 mg. %. Creatnine clearance is obtained by collecting a 24-hour sample of urine. Normal creatnine clearance is between 130 and 140 ml per minute.

CROHN'S DISEASE Another name for granulomatous colitis, after Dr. Burrill Crohn. Inflammatory bowel disease that may lead to ileostomy or removal of portions of the intestinal tract.

CYSTECTOMY Surgical removal of the urinary bladder.

CYSTOSCOPE An instrument with a light source and eye-piece that allows visualization of the urinary bladder.

CYSTOSCOPY Examination of the bladder with a cystoscope.

DECUBITUS Lying down. Often the term erroneously used for a pressure sore.

DEHISCENCE Separation of all layers of an incision, the "coming apart of."

DEHYDRATION The result of excessive water loss. It may result from inadequate fluid intake, vomiting, or other conditions.

DESCENDING COLON The portion of the colon on the left side of the body between the splenic flexure and the sigmoid colon (See Figure 4).

DILATE Stretch (distend) beyond normal size. Surgeons used to recommend that stomas be dilated to keep them open. This is no longer common practice.

DISTAL   Farthest away from the beginning or central point. Opposite of proximal.

DIVERSION   Variation or departure from the normal course, such as urinary or bowel diversion.

DIVERTICULUM   Little sac or outpouching in the walls of a canal or organ.

ELECTROLYTES   Normal components of body fluids, such as salt, potassium, etc. Electrolyte imbalance causes illness.

ENCRUSTATION   "Warty" looking, grey eruptions around the stoma. Usually associated with alkaline urine bathing the skin.

ENDOSCOPY   Procedure to visualize any cavity of the body with an instrument.

ENTERITIS   Inflammation of the intestine. Usually refers to the small intestine.

ENTEROSTOMAL THERAPIST   A registered nurse (if recently certified) with specialized training in the management of all types of stomas and draining wounds and the psychological needs specific to patients with such disorders. An ET must be graduated from an approved training school and should be certified by an examining board. (Nurses training was not required of the earliest practitioners who actually founded the profession. Some are still practicing today.)

EPIDERMIS   The outermost layer of skin.

EPITHELEAL   Cells that cover the internal and external surfaces of the body, including the lining of vessels and other small cavities, such as bladder epithelium.

EXCORIATION   Red, raw skin. Usually excoriation is the result of mechanical abrasion or fecal or urine burn.

EXSTROPHY OF THE BLADDER   A birth defect in which the bladder, "turned wrong side out" is exposed on the abdominal wall. (See discussion on p. 108)

FAMILIAL POLYPOSIS   A disease characterized by numerous polyps in the colon and rectum. Because it is a familial disease, all members of the family should be closely supervised. Early detection and removal of diseased organs is required to prevent malignancy.

FECES   Body wastes discharged through the anus, colostomy, or ileostomy. Stool.

FLATUS   Gas.

FISTULA   An abnormal opening between two hollow organs or between a hollow organ and the outside of the body.

GI SERIES   X-rays of the gastrointestinal tract

GRANULATION   Granular cells of new tissue that form on the surface of wounds and ulcers. May be part of the normal healing process or, in some cases, excessive accumulation of new tissue.

HERNIA   Protrusion or bulging of a loop or knuckle of an organ or tissue through a structure that usually contains it, such as an inguinal hernia or a parastomal hernia.

HIRSCHSPRUNG'S DISEASE   An intestinal defect characterized by the absence of ganglion nerves. (See discussion on p. 105).

HYDROCEPHALUS   (Hydro—water; cephalus—head.) An abnormal collection of cerebrospinal fluid in the brain. (See discussion on p. 110)

HYDRONEPHROSIS   (Hydro—water; nephro—kidney.) Enlargement of one or both kidneys caused by urine that has not passed freely to the outside of the body.

HYDROURETERONEPHROSIS   (Hydro—water; uretero—ureters that lead from the kidneys to the bladder; nephro—kidney.) Enlargement of one or both kidneys and one or both ureters, caused by urine that has not passed freely to the outside of the body.

ILEAL   Pertaining to the ileum or lower third of the small intestine.

ILEUM   The lower third of the small intestine.

ILEAL CONDUIT   An operation to divert urine away from a diseased or deformed bladder. A short segment of ileum is used as a conduit to transport urine from the ureters to the outside of the body. (See Figure 21) Also called a Bricker Loop, after Dr. Eugene Bricker, or ileal loop. Sometimes it is referred to as an "ileal bladder" (a misnomer because the conduit is not meant to contain urine), and sometimes an "ileostomy" (which causes confusion with fecal ileostomy).

ILEITIS   Inflammation of the ileum, also called regional enteritis, Crohn's disease, or regional ileitis.

ILEOCECAL VALVE   The low-pressure valve at the junction of the ileum and cecum that prevents the backing up of ileal contents.

ILEOSTOMY   Surgical opening into the ileum. (See Figure 10)

IMPERFORATE ANUS   The absence of an anal opening in the newborn. (See discussion on p. 104)

IMPOTENT   Inability to achieve or sustain an erection.

INCONTINENCE   Inability to control elimination of stool or urine.

IRRIGATION   An enema or wash-out of the colon to regulate passage of a stool.

IVP   Intravenous pyelogram. Medicine is injected into the veins, which permits visualization of the kidneys, ureters and bladder. On normal x-rays soft tissues are not visible.

JEJUNOSTOMY   A surgical opening into the jejunun.

JEJUNUM   The portion of the small intestine between the duodenum and the ileum.

KARAYA   By-product of the bark of a tree found in India. Refined it becomes karaya powder. Mixed with other substances it may be made into paste or wafers of varying consistency.

KARAYA GUM POWDER   A water-soluble powder used for healing or preventing excoriated skin

KUB   Abbreviation for kidney, ureters, bladder. The term refers to an x-ray taken of that portion of the body.

LATERAL   Pertaining to the right or left of the midline of the body. To one side.

LUMEN   Cavity or channel within a tube or tubular organ.

MALIGNANT   Characterized by abnormally rapid cellular reproduction. Refers to cancer or rapidly worsening disease.

MATURATION   The stage or process of becoming mature. When referring to human development it describes biological, physical, social, and psychological processes. When referring to a stoma, it describes the manner in which the intestine is turned back over itself. Failure to mature a stoma contributes to malfunction in ileostomies, and stenosis in other types of ostomies.

METASTASIS   Spreading of disease from one organ or body part to another.

MUCOUS FISTULA   An opening to the outside of the body from a defunctionalized or bypassed segment of small or large intestine. A mucous fistula is not connected to the fecal stream. It may secret mucus. It may shrivel and be hardly apparent.

MUCUS   Fluid secreted from cells or glands, that moistens membranes.

MYELOMENINGOCELE   Protrusion of spinal cord and covering through a defect in the bony spine. (See discussion on p. 110)

NASOGASTRIC TUBE   A tube inserted through the nose and threaded down into the stomach. Used to protect the bowel after intestinal surgery, or to relieve obstruction.

NEONATAL NECROTIZING ENTEROCOLITIS   A phenomenon that occurs most frequently in premature infants of low birthweight in which a segment of the bowel is necrotic (not living). An ileostomy may be a lifesaving measure. (See discussion on p. 103)

NEONATE   A newborn baby in the first two weeks of life.

NEPHROSTOMY   A surgical opening into the kidney, managed with a tube. (See Figure 15)

NEUROGENIC BLADDER   (Neuro—nerve; genus—origin.) A term that refers to bladder abnormality caused by nerve damage.

OSTOMATE   A person who has an ostomy.

OSTOMIST   The word preferred by the English and some other foreigners to describe a person who has an ostomy.

OSTOMY   Until recently a suffix. Now (at least among involved professionals, patients and caretakers), an accepted word used to discuss the various surgically created openings into the gastrointestinal or urinary systems.

PERINEAL   Pertaining to the perineum.

PERINEUM   The space between the anus and the genital organs. Often used in general conversation to describe the area between the legs.

PERISTALSIS   A squeezing rythmic motion found in the alimentary canal and the ureters in the urinary tract.

pH   Indicator of acidity or alkalinity—frequently used in discussion of urinary pH. Uninfected urine usually is on the acid side of neutral. Bacteria do not grow well in acid urine, but thrive in alkaline urine. Patients with urinary conduits may be given medication, diet, or advice to drink cranberry juice to acidify their urine.

POSTERIOR   In back of or back part of.

PROCTOSCOPY   Visual examination of the rectum by means of a hollow instrument, a proctoscope.

PROJECTILE VOMITING   The forceful ejection of vomit, distinguishable from spitting up or vomiting associated with minor upsets. Vomit is also referred to as emesis.

PROLAPSE   A falling down of an organ or part. In ostomy nomenclature, prolapse refers to an abnormal lengthening of the bowel through the stoma.

PROSTHESIS   An artificial device used to replace a missing limb or body part.

PROXIMAL   Nearest the point of attachment or origin. Opposite of distal.

PURULENT   Consisting of pus, infected.

REFLUX   A flowing back. Reflux of urine from the bladder back up to the kidney is abnormal.

REGIONAL ENTERITIS   See ileitis.

RESECTION   Surgical removal or excision.

RESIDUAL URINE   Urine left behind in bladder or intestinal conduit. This is an undesirable condition because pooling of urine invites bacterial overgrowth and infection.

RETRACTION   The act of drawing back. Some stomas retract into the body making management very difficult.

REVISION   Surgical relocation of the stoma to a new site or reconstruction of the stoma at the present site.

SIGMOIDOSCOPY   Visual examination of the rectum and lower part of sigmoid colon with a sigmoidoscope.

SKIN BARRIER   The term commonly used to describe synthetic gelatinous material that is tacky enough to adhere to the skin and protects skin from external sources of irritation. Plastic films applied as sprays, wipes, or paint-ons may also be called skin barriers. Stomahesive, Reliaseal and Skin-Prep are skin barriers. A karaya washer is also referred to by some as a skin barrier.

SKIN CEMENT   Preparation in tube, spray can, or container with applicator, used to affix ostomy appliances to skin.

SOLVENT   Fluid used to remove cement and adhesive residue from skin and appliance.

SPHINCTER   A ring-like muscle that is able to open and close. Bowel and bladder control depend upon effective sphincter control.

SPINA BIFIDA   A defect in the bony spine. (See discussion on p. 110)

STENOSIS   Narrowing of a passageway or opening. Narrowing or excessive tightness of the stoma that may cause obstruction.

STOMA   Mouth. In ostomy nomenclature it is commonly used when referring to the end of the ureter, ileum, or colon that is seen coming through the skin.

STRICTURE   Narrowing.

TRAUMA   Physical injury caused by a mechanical force, as a blow, twist, knife, or bullet. Psychological trauma is an injury to the subconscious mind by emotional shock.

ULCERATIVE COLITIS   Inflammation of the colon characterized by such symptoms as bloody stools, diarrhea, and abdominal cramps. (See discussion on p. 105)

UMBILICUS   Pertaining to the navel.

URETER   Tube leading from the kidney to the bladder.

URETEROSTOMY   A surgical opening into the ureter. (See Figures 17, 18)

URINARY DIVERSION   Any one of a number of surgical procedures that divert urine from its normal course of flow.

URINARY TRACT   The system in the body comprised of the kidneys, ureters, bladder, and urethra. In the male the reproductive system is intimately connected to the urinary tract.

URODYNAMICS   The study of the act of voiding and the function of the urinary system in motion.

VESICOSTOMY   Surgical opening into the bladder. (See Figure 19)

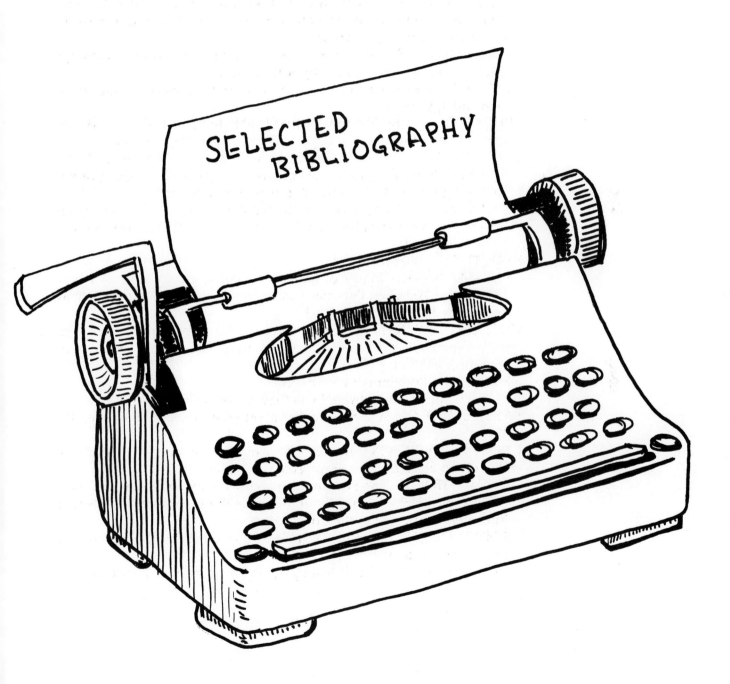

A selected bibliography

The following titles are offered for those who are interested in further reading. They were selected from a more comprehensive list of references that is available from the author.

Arnstein, Helene S.: 1960. *What to Tell Your Child*. New York, Bobbs-Merrill.

Azarnoff, P., and Flegal, S.: 1975. *A Pediatric Play Program*. Springfield, IL, Charles C. Thomas.

Barnard, K.: 1975. *A Program Of Stimulation For Infants Born Prematurely*. Seattle, WA, Univ. of Washington Press.

Belgum, D.C.: 1974. *What Can I Do About The Part Of Me I Don't Like?* Minneapolis, MN, Augsberg Publishing House.

Bettleheim, B.: 1972. "How Do You Help a Child Who Has a Physical Handicap?" *Ladies Home Journal* 89:34-35.

Brazelton, T. Berry: 1981. *On Becoming A Family: The Growth of Attachment*. New York, Delacorte Press.

Briggs, Dorothy: 1970. *Your Child's Self-Esteem*. Garden City, New York, Doubleday & Company, Inc.

Buscaglia, Leo (ed.): 1975. *The Disabled And Their Parents: A Counseling Challenge*. Thorofare, NJ, Charles B. Slack.

(The) Children's Hospital Medical Center Health Education Dept.: 1970. *Your Child and Ileal Conduit Surgery*. Springfield, IL, C. R. Thomas.

Cole, K. C.: 1980. *What Only A Mother Can Tell You About Having A Baby*. Garden City, NY, Anchor Press.

Coopersmith, S.: 1967. *The Antecedents of Self-Esteem*. San Francisco, CA, W. H. Freeman.

Erikson, E. H.: 1963. *Childhood and Society*. 2nd ed., New York, W. W. Norton.

Erikson, E. H.: 1968. *Identity, Youth And Crisis*. New York, W. W. Norton.

Faber, Adele, and Mazlish, Elaine: 1974. *Liberated Parents, Liberated Children*, New York, Grosset & Dunlap.

Ginott, Haim: 1969. *Between Parent And Child*. New York, Macmillan.

Gordon, T.: 1970. *Parent Effectiveness Training*. New York, Peter Wyden.

Klaus, M. H. and Kennell, J. H.: 1976. *Maternal-Infant Bonding*. St. Louis, MO, C. V. Mosby.

McCollum, A.: 1975. *Coping With Prolonged Health Impairment In Your Child*. Boston, Little, Brown, and Co.

Murphy, L. B., and Moriarity, A. E.: 1976. *Vulnerability, Coping and Growth—From Infancy to Adolescence*, New Haven, CT, Yale University Press.

Petrillo, M. and Sanger, S.: 1972. *Emotional Care of Hospitalized Children.* Philadelphia, J. B. Lippincott Co.

Pogrebin, L. D.: 1980. *Growing Up Free: Raising Your Child In the '80s.* New York, McGraw-Hill.

Salk, Lee: 1972. *What Every Child Would Like His Parents to Know.* New York, David McKay.

Satir, Virginia: 1972. *Peoplemaking.* Palo Alto, CA., Science and Behavior Books, Inc.

Steele, S. (ed): 1971. *Nursing Care Of The Child With Long-Term Illness.* New York, Appleton-Century Crafts.

Trachtenberg, Inge: 1978. *My Daughter, My Son.* New York, Summit Books.

Weiss, Louise: 1977. *Access To The World.* New York, Chatham Square Press.

Dear Parents:

Soon you will become experts in the care of your children's ostomies. You will come up with new solutions to old problems and inventive ideas that save energy, and money. We hope you'll take the time to share them with other parents.

We also welcome your comments after reading this book. Thank you for taking the time.

Katherine Jeter
c/o Bull Publishing Co.
P.O. Box 208
Palo Alto, CA 94302

Appendix A

A dietician will have information, recipes and printed material to help you plan for your children's nutritional needs. The following highlights and diets are offered to answer your initial questions.

FOOD HIGHLIGHTS FOR OSTOMATES

Easily digested foods:
- Bouillon
- Cream soups
- Macaroni or noodles
- Potatoes, baked or mashed
- Refined rice

Potassium-rich foods:
- Bananas
- Cocoa
- Colas
- Dried fruits
- Flavored meat extract
- Grapefruit
- Molasses
- Rye crackers
- Oranges
- Tea
- Tomatoes

Sodium-rich foods:
- Bacon
- Butter
- Crackers
- Dried beef
- Mayonnaise
- Salmon and tuna
- Salt
- Snack Foods—chips, etc.
- Mustard
- Pretzels

Gas-producing foods:
- Cabbage and cabbage family
- Asparagus
- Broccoli
- Cucumbers
- Dried beans
- Eggs
- Fish
- Onions
- Radishes

Hard-to-digest foods that may cause obstruction or abdominal discomfort:

Celery	Olives
Coconut	Peppers
Corn on the cob	Pickles
Chinese vegetables	Pineapple
Fresh grapes	Popcorn
Fried foods	Seeds
Mushrooms	Whole grain cereals
Nuts	

Remedies for dehydration:

1. Coca-cola plus one tsp. salt (stir bubbles out first)
2. One glass water with one tsp. baking soda
3. Three cups tea and sugar
4. Gatorade, Energade, Electrolytes Plus

NOTE: Lactose intolerance is not uncommon. Commonly consumed foods with lactose are:

Milk and milk products—cheese, margarine, sherbet, yogurt
Prepared mixes, cereals, soups, gravies, instant drinks

Appendix B

LOW RESIDUE DIET

Beverages:
    *Milk, limited to one pint (as such or in cooking), boiled if necessary
    Coffee
    Tea
    Postum

    All others excluded

Breads:
    Enriched toasted white bread
    Plain white crackers
    Melba toast

    All others excluded

Cereals:
    Cooked cream of wheat
    Farina
    Cream of rice
    Cornmeal
    Hominy grits

    All others excluded

Desserts:
    Clear flavored gelatin and rennet desserts
    Custard
    Plain puddings
    Fruit whips (from allowed fruits)
    Ice cream
    Sherbets
    Plain cakes
    Plain cookies

    Nuts, coconut, raisins, rich pastries and desserts excluded

*Milk and milk products may not be tolerated well by some children.

Fats:

Butter and margarine
Cream in moderation

All others excluded

Fruits:

Bananas
Canned peaches
Pears
Applesauce

Other fruits strained
Strained fruit juices

Canned or fresh pineapple, berries, figs, raw fruits except bananas are excluded

Meats, egg, and cheeses:

Tender beef	Veal
Lamb	Chicken
Turkey	Liver
White fish	Crisp bacon
Tender lean roast pork	Oysters
Sweetbreads and brains	Salmon
Tuna	Cream cheese
Cottage cheese	Mild chedder cheese
Eggs any way except fried	(combined with other foods)

All cured and highly seasoned meats, any meat that has a tough fiber or gristle, and fried foods are excluded

Soups:

Any strained soup made from foods allowed
All others excluded

Vegetables:

All tender cooked or canned strained asparagus, carrots, beets, young peas, young snap beans, spinach, squash
White and sweet potatoes, without skins

All other vegetables strained
Tomato juice

All gaseous vegetables, raw or cooked, such as broccoli, brussel sprouts, cabbage, corn, turnips, cauliflower, cucumbers, green peppers, onions, radishes, and sauerkraut, all other raw vegetables, and dried peas and beans are excluded

Miscellaneous:

Salt and sugar in moderation	Cocoa
Cream sauces	Honey
Jelly	
Hard candy	

Pepper, highly seasoned foods, pickles, relishes, jams, nuts, olives, popcorn, and potato chips are excluded

Appendix C

ACID-ASH DIET*

Allowed:

    Breads   Oysters

    Cereals   Pastries

    Eggs   Poultry

    Fish   Puddings

    Meat

Neutral Ash Food Allowed:

    Butter   Sugar

    Cream   Tapioca

Milk, fruits, and vegetables are basically alkaline-ash but the following fruits and vegetables are permissible on an acid-ash diet:

Cranberries and cranberry juice	Plums
Cherry juice	Prunes
Grape juice	Fresh peaches
Fresh pears	Raspberry juice
Grapes	Watermelon

Asparagus	Fresh peas
Cauliflower	Pumpkin
Fresh string beans	Squash
Corn	Turnips
Mushrooms	

An acid-ash diet alone or in combination with urinary acidifiers may reduce odor and the alkalinity of urine that has been a problem to many children with urostomies. Do not make any dietary modification without consulting your physician.

---

*Food list taken from *Nursing Care of Patients with Urologic Diseases* (4th Ed.), C. V. Mosby, by Chester Winter, M.D. and Alice Morel, R.N.

Appendix D

Clean Intermittent Bladder Catheterization

An 8 Fr. or 10 Fr. catheter is recommended.

PROCEDURE

1. Wash hands with soap and water.
2. Clean perineal area with soap and water or disposable wipes. (Wet-Ones are convenient to carry in a pocket or purse.)
3. Gently insert catheter into urethra until the urine flows.
4. Drain bladder completely.
5. Remove catheter slowly.
6. Wash hands and catheter simultaneously. Rinse. Replace catheter in clean container.

Recommended containers for carrying catheter and cleansing wipes:
 Small cosmetic pouch
 Tobacco pouch
 Plastic cigarette package holder

Some urologists wish catheters to be washed in Hibiclens or other urinary disinfectants and stored in aluminum foil between use.

Kathleen Hannigan, RN, of the John F. Kennedy Institute in Baltimore, uses a teaching doll and a mirror to prepare preschoolers for doing their own catheterization. She seats the doll in front of the child and the child first uses the mirror to guide the catheter into the doll's urethra. Kathleen finds that a mental age of five is necessary to use this method. Before that it is not possible for children to understand that the mirror image is their own.

It has been recommended that a long-handled plastic dental mirror be taped to the catheter, well away from the portion to be inserted in the urethra, to facilitate positioning of the catheter in the urethra instead of the vagina in young girls.

For older girls, Dr. Larrian Gillespie of California suggests that they put a finger into the vagina and guide the catheter along that finger into the opening above it, the urethra.

GRAPHIC GLOSSARY AND COLORING SECTION

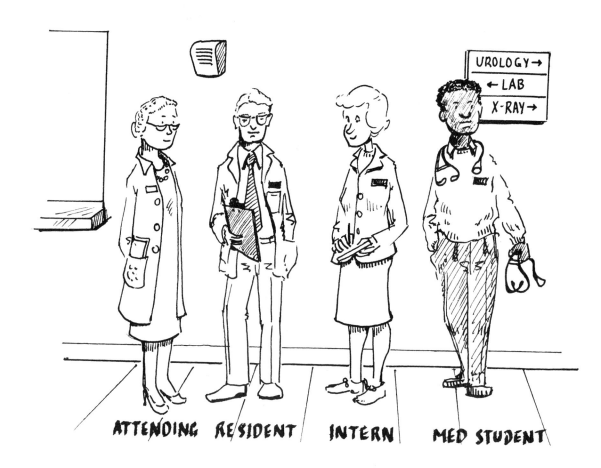

ATTENDING RESIDENT INTERN MED STUDENT

ATTENDING	An attending is a physician on the staff. Attendings are "in charge" in a teaching hospital.
RESIDENT	A resident is a physician who is studying a specialty such as gastroenterology, pediatrics, surgery, or urology. Chief residents are in their final year of training in their specialty.
INTERN	An internship of one year is served immediately following graduation from medical school. Interns work very hard.
MEDICAL STUDENTS	Medical students study medicine for four years in classrooms, hospitals, and outpatient settings.

NURSES ...

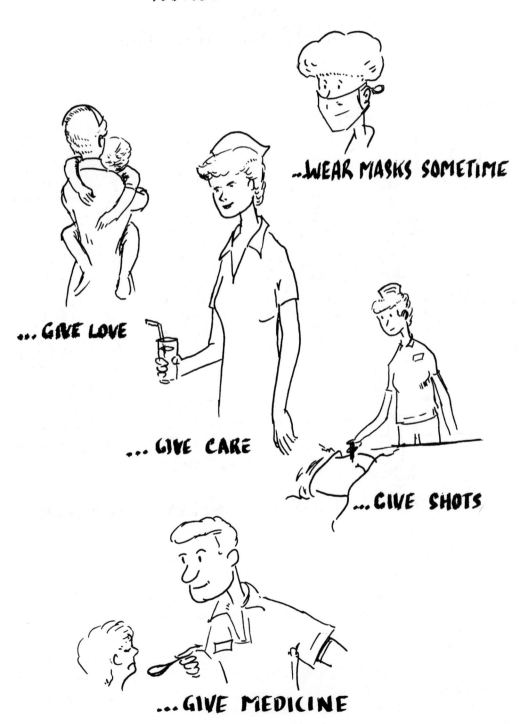

...WEAR MASKS SOMETIME

... GIVE LOVE

... GIVE CARE

...GIVE SHOTS

...GIVE MEDICINE

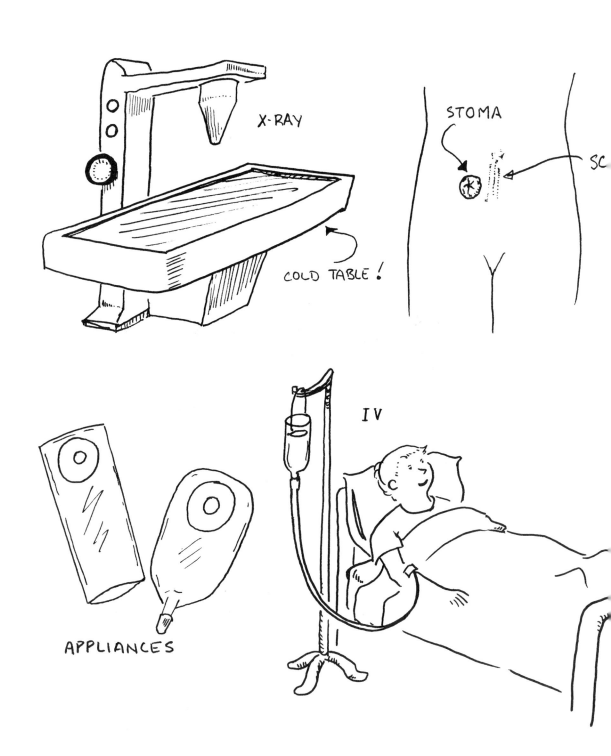

X-RAY

COLD TABLE!

STOMA

SC

APPLIANCES

IV

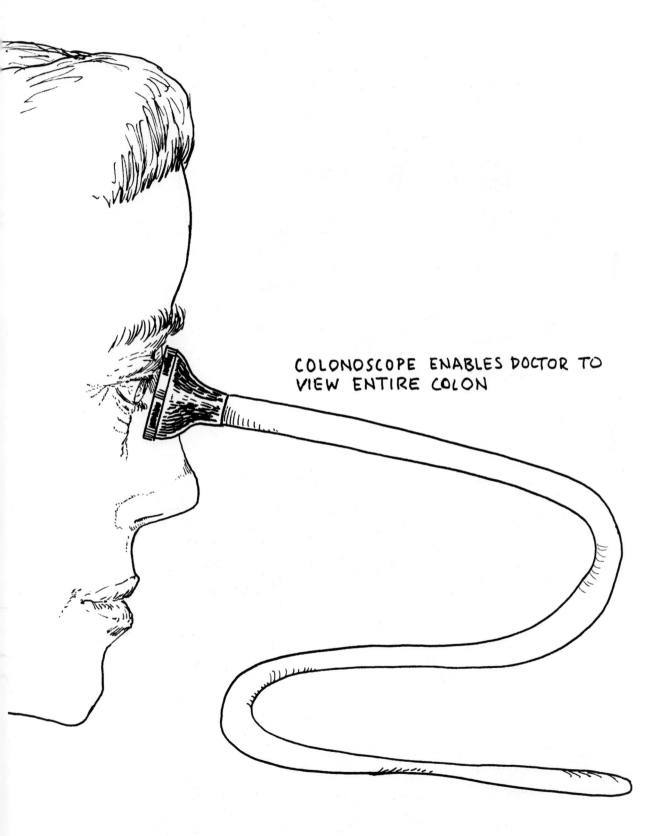

COLONOSCOPE ENABLES DOCTOR TO
VIEW ENTIRE COLON

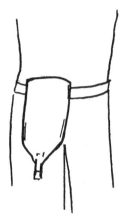

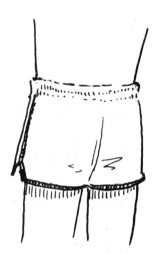

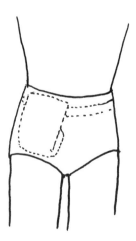

The following drawings are for children, mothers fathers and care givers to draw in stoma sites, appliances, anatomical parts of the body, etc. as a teaching and learning aide.

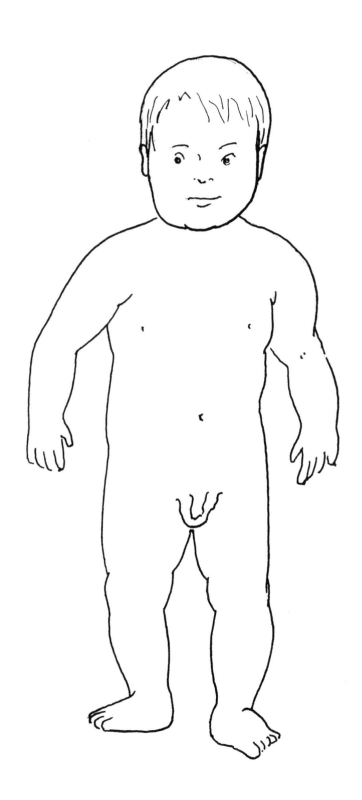

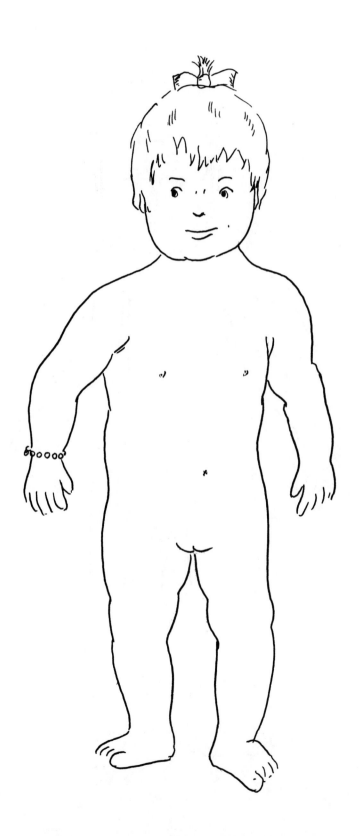

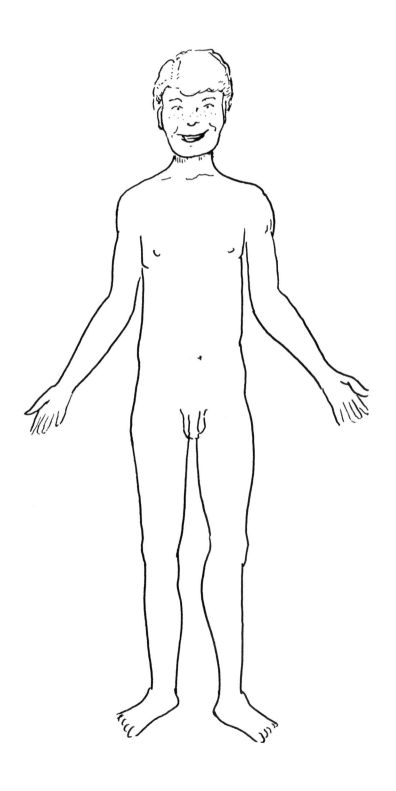

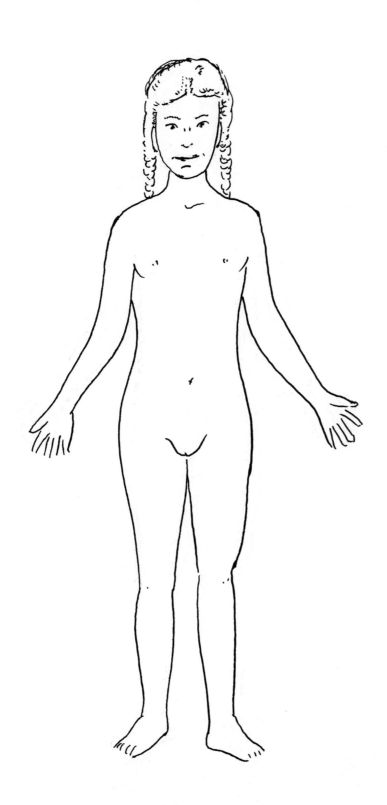

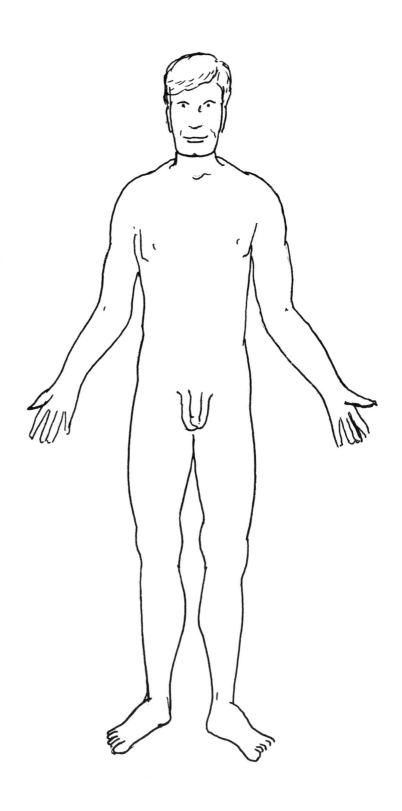

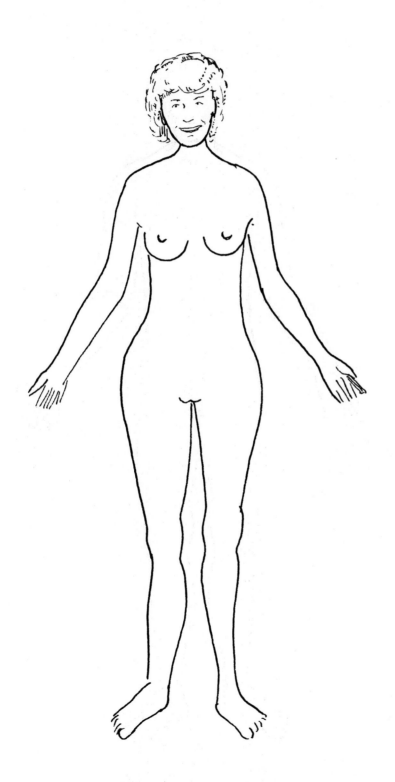

Index

Notes

Notes